Contents

THE
YIN YANG
GUIDE TO
WEIGHT LOSS

Lose weight through the ancient Chinese
philosophy of Yin and Yang

LILY LI HUA

JOHN BLAKE

Published by John Blake Publishing,
3 Bramber Court, 2 Bramber Road,
London W14 9PB, England

www.johnblakebooks.com

www.facebook.com/johnblakebooks ▪
twitter.com/jblakebooks ▪

This edition published in 2017

ISBN: 978 1 78606 829 3

British Library Cataloguing-in-Publication Data:

A catalogue record for this book is available from the British Library.

Design by www.envydesign.co.uk

Printed and bound in Great Britain by Clays Ltd, St Ives plc

1 3 5 7 9 10 8 6 4 2

Papers used by John Blake Publishing are natural, recyclable products
made from wood grown in sustainable forests. The manufacturing processes
conform to the environmental regulations of the country of origin.

Every attempt has been made to contact the relevant copyright-holders,
but some were unobtainable. We would be grateful if the appropriate people
could contact us.

John Blake Publishing is an imprint of Bonnier Publishing
www.bonnierpublishing.com

Foreword

Maintaining a healthy weight helps you to live a long, happy and healthy life. I have written this book to share with you the approach to diet and lifestyle which enables the Chinese to live long healthy lives whilst remaining slim, active and energetic up to old age.

Slimming is not just a young person's phenomenon; it concerns everyone, regardless of age or gender. Everybody should do everything in their power to live a healthier lifestyle.

Rarely do you hear someone question the decision to be slimmer and healthier, no one asks, 'Why do you want to be slim?' The common standard of beauty in society is that of the slim and healthy individual, who doesn't suffer from the many health conditions associated with weight gain or obesity; someone who appears to be fit and confident. It follows that we should do everything we can to pursue a healthier lifestyle.

People often ask me to help them become slim. Most people want to be slim but don't want to use slimming medicines, undergo surgery or any other invasive procedures. But people find it hard to continually measure or keep track of their daily intake of fat, sugar, carbohydrates, etc. to ensure a balanced diet. Calorie counting can often prove stressful and time consuming. Finance is often the biggest issue – not everyone can afford an expert team of dietitians, nutritionists or personal trainers. Slimming should be easy, enjoyable, and manageable and should fit naturally into your everyday life.

Many of my patients have talked to me about the difficulties they have experienced in losing weight. I have listened to every single one of you and understood perfectly. This book, which sets out the slimming secrets of Imperial China, is my response and can help put you on a path to a slimmer and healthier lifestyle.

China and the Chinese are considered to be one of the world's slimmest nations. A remarkably high percentage of the population is slim, compared to the rest of the world. People often ask what is the secret behind the good health and wellbeing enjoyed by the Chinese; the people are energetic, they work hard and enjoy food. Daily you see groups of people in the parks or public spaces practicing martial arts, running or dancing; most of this in the early morning around 5.00 am or in the evening after supper. This is how life should be.

Living naturally is the Chinese secret to slimming, the history of which dates back 3,000 years. Slimming was used to maintain good health and treat illness. The

Chinese believe that life should be natural and aligned with nature, nature in this case means Yin and Yang balance. This, they believed would help to keep you slim and healthy. If you incorporate the principles of Yin and Yang in your daily life, you can lose as much weight as you desire and you will be in control of your health and wellbeing.

The book tells you how the Chinese approach slimming and wellness on a daily basis; and it provides recipes and exercises. You can choose to learn bit by bit, day by day, until you can fully incorporate this approach into your everyday life. As you follow my guidance, you will start to notice the benefits, and not only for slimming but to revolutionise your energy, happiness and health.

The enormous benefits of adopting the Chinese approach to diet and lifestyle will transform your health and wellbeing, and not only you but future generations too.

I wish you success as you start this journey. Take control of your own health.

CHAPTER 1

My Motivation for Writing This Book

England is my second home and a wonderful country to live in. I have been a Londoner for 18 years and love living here. The environment is beautiful and life is interesting, rich in culture and history. The quality of life is good with free education, free health care, and respect for equality and diversity.

My lifetime's work is to help people with their health and wellbeing. Traditional Chinese Medicine has been my family's business dating back several generations and I have been steeped in it since I was a child. In the past 30 years, I have worked very hard to solve the health problems and issues of wellbeing presented by my patients.

It is very important to me to understand in an academic sense the differences between Chinese and Western medicine. Westerners are very interested in Traditional

Chinese Medicine – they value and trust this ancient and tried medical system. It is natural, effective and without side effects. This interest inspired me to establish my own Traditional Chinese Medicine business in London

In my 15 years as a practitioner of Traditional Chinese medicine and acupuncture in London, my patients have presented me with a whole range of health conditions. But I soon found something striking – more and more people were experiencing problems of weight gain leading to serious health problems. These problems, linked to the modern way of living, include heart disease, diabetes, stroke, and cancer. These conditions can be fatal or condemn people to a life of ill health.

Many had unsuccessfully tried to lose excess weight, using dietary supplements or medications. It was incredibly satisfying for me to find I could make a real difference in helping people resolve these dietary and health issues by simply applying the principles of Yin and Yang balance to their diet and lifestyle – enabling them to lose weight and achieve wellbeing in a few steps. Since then I have specialised in weight management.

Treating these conditions with Western medicine is costly and puts a lot of pressure on the National Health Service, both financially and in terms of staff. I believe that educating people about the Chinese philosophy of diet and lifestyle will enable them to lead healthier lives and prevent many of these serious illnesses.

I have read widely on Chinese diet and philosophy. Yet none of these books talk in-depth about how Chinese people stay slim. A key point is that the Chinese treat their bodies holistically. This is one of the fundamental principles of Yin and Yang balance. In this book, I will introduce you to the secrets of Chinese slimming – secrets which you can easily adopt and practice in your daily life.

In the course of my professional life I have successfully helped many people lose weight and stay slim. I have been interviewed on TV and by national newspapers and have given free lessons to educate people about Chinese medicine, giving them an insight into and knowledge of its 3,000-year history.

This book is essentially my heartfelt gift to say thank you to the people I have met and in appreciation of the life I enjoy in this country. This is my contribution to helping to ensure we have a healthier, slimmer and happier nation

CHAPTER 2

The Chinese Way of Life

Today, most people wish to be slim. Not only is being slim in fashion, people understand its importance in maintaining good health and wellbeing. The question is: How do we get slim and stay slim?

There are many obstacles to becoming slim. People do not have the time to cook healthy food regularly at home. The food industry produces mostly processed and fast food, often high in sugar and salt – not only is it unhealthy, it causes weight gain. Health experts advise that individuals calculate daily nutritional intake such as fat, sugar, proteins, carbohydrate, cholesterol, vitamins, fibre, iron, etc. to keep our diet on track. It is difficult to keep track of this and incorporate it into our busy, pressured, working lives. Some people eat out frequently as an alternative to eating junk or fast food.

We know that unhealthy eating and obesity is the root cause of many of society's ills –obesity, high blood pressure, heart problems, diabetes and cancers, etc. In the face of this, eating healthily and maintaining a healthy weight is a priority.

We all know Chinese people are slim and love eating. 'Have you had your meals?' (Ni chi fan le ma?) is the equivalent of the English greeting 'How are you?' How do the Chinese manage to combine their love of food and eating with staying slim – a seeming contradiction.

The answer lies in the oriental philosophy of diet. The Chinese believe that wellbeing comes from what we eat. This approach to food and diet has been tried and tested over the last 2,000 years. Many ancient Chinese philosophers and naturalists have researched and studied diet, wellbeing and good health. Their books record these research findings and have guided us down the generations on how to keep healthy and prevent disease. Those writings also refer to slimming and fitness, and their findings are as relevant today as they were then.

Interestingly, throughout the Qing Dynasty (1644-1912), ruling Emperors placed great emphasis on finding the secrets of longevity. In response, the central government of the time developed a healthcare education system and established numerous academic organisations to research and develop Traditional Chinese Medicine, wellbeing, diet, martial arts and Chinese tea. Today, in China, Traditional Chinese Medicine continues to be as popular as ever and research continues into the Chinese lifestyle, philosophy and medicine. Many texts have been handed down recording our ancestors' knowledge and practices, and these have been found to be still relevant today (there is an old Chinese saying: 'Sickness comes from the mouth').

Diet is unquestionably related to health. A healthy diet equals being slim and healthy. Being slim lowers the risk of developing the illnesses of modern life. I have lived in England for 18 years. My partner is English. We have several differences in lifestyle. I have always been slim while he was overweight when we met. Since adopting the Chinese way of eating and living he has become slim.

So, what is the secret of the Chinese approach to slimming?

People live very simple lives in China. Perhaps a simple life is an adventure, more spontaneous, healthier and less stressful. I will give you examples of their lifestyle throughout this book. You will be interested to see that they live according to their own natural rhythm, eating vegetables, fruit, meat, sometimes drinking rice wine and exercising to meet the needs of their body.

Their lives are in tune with their bodies, maintaining physical activity in response to the needs of their body and depending on the amount of time they have. Exercise is never forced. They are following their body in Yin and Yang balance. Very importantly, they all have a very strong in-depth knowledge of the Chinese philosophy of healthy eating and living.

Journalist Dan Buettner, in partnership with National Geographic, during more than five years of on-site investigation of blue zones (places in the world where people live longer and healthier lives than anywhere else on Earth), found longevity and good health depended on four important facts:

- Healthy, organic food (plenty of vegetables, fruits, fish and nuts. Low on meat, sugar, fat and toxic, processed foods)
- As stress free a life as possible
- Regular exercise
- Community skills, caring and being cared for, respect for others and receiving respect in return

Several of these blue zones exist, and in each of these places people routinely live to ninety or even one hundred years. And they aren't just living long lives either – these people are living healthy lives – without medication or disability. His pioneering approach is similar to the Chinese philosophy on diet and lifestyle.

CHAPTER 3

The Philosophy of Yin and Yang

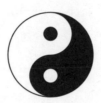

The Yin and Yang (i.e. taijitu symbol) shows a balance between two opposites with a portion of the opposite element in each section. In Taoist metaphysics, distinctions between good and bad, along with other dichotomous moral judgments, are perceptual, not real; so, the duality of Yin and Yang is an indivisible whole. The philosophy of Yin and Yang is perhaps the most known and documented concept within Taoism.

The definition of Yin and Yang is: two halves that together complete a whole. Yin and Yang are also the starting point for change. When something is whole, by definition it is unchanging and complete. When you split something into two halves – Yin and Yang, it upsets the equilibrium of wholeness. This starts both halves chasing after each other as they seek a new balance with each other.

The word Yin means 'female side' and is represented by a female symbol. Yang means 'male side' and is represented by a male symbol. Different symbols such as 'moon' versus 'sun' are used to explain this. I have shown the commonly used symbol of Yin and Yang as a pair.

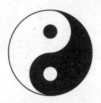

Yin and Yang is the concept of duality forming a whole. We encounter examples of Yin and Yang every day – e.g. night (Yin) and day (Yang); sad (Yin) and happy (Yang). Over thousands of years, a number of Yin and Yang classification systems have been developed.

The symbol for Yin and Yang is called the Taijitu. In the West it is generally referred to as the Yin and Yang symbol. The Taijitu symbol has been found in more than one culture and over the years has come to represent Taoism.

Yin and Yang works to the rules of nature and has been used widely in Chinese thought, culture, astrology, geography, health, living, etc. The principles of Yin and Yang were developed originally by the philosopher Laozi. He and later philosophers decreed that all things should be seen as part of a whole. No entity can ever be isolated from its relationship to other entities; nothing can exist in and of itself, there are no absolutes. Yin and Yang must, necessarily, contain within themselves the possibility of opposition and change.

I have sometimes found a similar philosophy in the West, example, it is not unusual to hear someone say 'think positively, don't think negatively'. Here the positive and negative function as a pair, positive is Yang, negative is Yin.

The philosophy of Yin and Yang is not easy to understand so I have set out below a table showing some examples of Yin and Yang as they occur in daily life.

Yin Symbol	Yang Symbol
Moon	Sun
Female	Male
Night	Day
Back	Front
Inside	Outside
Poor	Rich
Dark	Red
Green	Yellow
White	Black
Bitter	Sweet
Sad	Happy
Relaxed	Active
Calm	Anxious
Vegetables	Meat
Cold	Hot

Yin and Yang philosophy is illustrated with the traditional 3,000-year-old Chinese Taoist symbol shown below and now widely recognised. The big circle represents the universe and the small circle represents the human body divided into Yin and Yang.

The universe and human body have the same essence and attributes. They obey the same rules of development. It is considered that humans should adapt to nature and obey the laws of nature. Thus Yin and Yang create each other, control each other and transform into each other. Because of the pervasive influence of Yin and Yang theory on Chinese thought and culture, the Chinese understand and explain things differently.

For example, 24 hours is a whole day – day is white, night is black and together they create a circle. That is the natural way of life on earth. People work in the day and sleep at night. That is the human life circle. The human body needs to obey change in the natural earth.

There needs to be a balance between hours worked and time spent resting. If you work too much, Yang energy is used up; automatically this reduces Yin energy. The laws of nature suggest Yin and Yang are controlling each other.

Human behaviour should follow changes in the environment. When the weather is hot, warm air flowing through the body will cause the body temperature to rise, resulting in excess Yang energy. People should eat more cold food and drink cold water to redress the balance.

When the human body suffers excessive coldness, an overload of Yin will also cause an imbalance. People should eat more hot food, drink hot water and let their skin absorb more sunshine to get in and Yang balance again.

When pollution levels are high, your body will get toxins through the air flow to the body. It can gradually damage the Yin and Yang balance – this can affect some organs or the whole body system, especially the function of the lungs and liver. It can also reduce the function of the immune system.

Environment can help restore balance to the body. For example, when you are exhausted through work or too much thinking, walk around an open-air space such as a garden, park, along the coast or in the mountains. The warm climate will boost Yang energy. Cold climate will boost Yin energy

Nature has given us a sense of what is good to drink. Organic food is better for the body as it is grown naturally without chemicals. When you eat organic food, your body is comfortable, foods easily digested, it is less toxic and uses less energy.

So the philosophy of Yin and Yang balance is connected to natural law and the environment this has an impact on the body.

24-Hour Cycle

The 24 hour daily cycle of working, sleeping, eating and drinking are fixed natural laws. Activities (e.g. exercise) can be flexible. Yang will provide energy for all your functions and activity, Yin will provide energy to maintain, repair and nourish. This pairing of Yin and Yang balance can change. For instance when your Yin is low, say through hard work, to rebalance you can lower your Yang or raise your Yin by reducing your work.

For example, if you are overworked it causes Yang deficiency and leads to a Yin and Yang imbalance. You can suffer from uncomfortable to chronic tiredness or sickness. In this situation, how can you rebalance your Yang and Yang energy? There are several different ways that can help you:

- Eating Yang energy food, such as meat, black mushroom, black fungus, tofu, nuts. Also selected vegetables, fruits and teas containing a high level of Yang energy.
- Reducing your activity to restore your Yin energy. You can take a rest or practice general meditation; conserve your energy
- Getting energy through activities that need less energy
- You can listen to music, cook, be socially active or take exercise to increase Yang energy.

When you haven't slept or rested well, your body's Yang energy will be low and Yin energy high. The balance will be lost, and you will feel tired and bloated. To rebalance your Yin and Yang energy try the following:

- Boost Yang energy by reducing sleep time immediately.

- Boost Yang energy through physical activity or exercise
- Reduce foods that have Yin energy and increase those with Yang energy, and reduce portion size

When you have too much mental activity it causes both Yang and Yin energy to be lowered. You can raise your energy by taking a rest, having regular exercise and relaxing. Choose foods that are both high in Yin and Yang, such as black mushroom, black fungus, tofu, nuts, kiwis, oranges, bananas and strawberries as these increase brain power and strength.

If you have been eating too much, your Yang energy level is low due to the body using energy to digest. You can balance Yin and Yang by reducing your food; try to stay 30% hungry.

You cannot easily change the natural laws governing the body's wellbeing – only on occasion. If you force change to this cycle, the result is discomfort, pain, sleeplessness, bloating, weight gain, etc. If the body is forced to suddenly or permanently abandon these natural laws due to stress, pressure or injuries, you will suffer from serious illness and your life may even be in danger.

Chinese wellbeing is the Yin and Yang balance. In the West people often say 'please look after yourself', and we are aiming for the same goal. The Chinese method is more accurate through Yin and Yang balance philosophy. The Western method to health and happiness is without rules for daily life, it doesn't accurately measure your work life balance. You may look ok but have underlying health problems.

In China and the West we are concerned for our wellbeing, the human body needs discipline. I recently had a conversation with a client who is a personal trainer and health and fitness consultant. We talked about how our bodies are similar to a car and has its own life span. If you care about it you will maintain it, change the oil, and drive it carefully. It will function well, look good and have a long life. That same principle applies to our body. In the 24 hour cycle, your body needs regular work, sleep, exercise and social activities. With that you will be healthy, energetic and maintain a healthy weight.

Sadly in the West, people, especially those working in banking, finance and IT sectors, work 10-12 hours per day and also weekends. The day is only 24 hours long which leaves little time for exercise, physical activity, eating and sleeping. This lifestyle does not obey the body's natural laws of Yin and Yang balance, and their health is in danger of being damaged.

Patients sometimes tell me 'there is no gym near my office', or 'my energy is low after a long day's work', or 'after the gym I feel more tired and exhausted'. In this case, remember that you don't have to go to the gym. Instead walk, run, play tennis or cycle. When you are tired, listen to music, work in the garden, go out with friends or family or engage in other social activities – all of which help the body function better in terms of Yin and Yang balance. Engage in these activities regularly and your body will function better than if you didn't. Activities are flexible, they can be combined with exercise. When you do this you will work more efficiently and think faster. In Chinese terms, you will have Yin and Yang balance. In Western terms you will enjoy a balanced mind, body and soul.

I set out below how to change your lifestyle so that it follows the body's natural 24 hour cycle. I have given you several stages so that you can reach your goal in terms of wellbeing and weight loss:

- Follow the philosophy of Yin and Yang balance
- Follow the A, B, C, D daily routine in Chapter 7
- Diet – follow the principles of Yin and Yang balance

To lose weight, you should leave the table a little hungry and take exercise. Do not force your body to do more exercise than your body tells you. The Chinese exercise daily – try to adopt this practice when you can.

Physical activity every day, including exercise, is vital for good health. In the West you constantly hear that 'exercise is good for you' and there is an old Chinese saying 'walk a hundred footsteps after dinner, you will live to be 99 years old'.

The Chinese prefer to do physical activities, including exercise, in the open (in parks, fields, close to an ancient tree, by the riverbank or lake) as close to nature as possible.

The benefits of being outdoors include fresh air and oxygen, and a relaxing environment. Chinese philosophy considers that doing activity outdoors causes the body's

Qi (vital energy) to flow faster and more regularly, to detox and be ready for work, helping the mind to focus more easily.

The Chinese do their physical activity in the morning before breakfast to increase Yang energy levels for the whole day. They drink water on an empty stomach, then practice martial arts e.g. Qigong, Taijiquan, or go walking, running, dancing, etc.

They take two hours for lunch to include eating, activities and a nap. Physical activities recharge Yin and Yang energy in the body. This traditional system has been developed to meet the needs of the body. After a morning's work, the body needs to relax.

At the end of the day in China, different activities are undertaken. It is time to relax, help the mind switch off and release the stress of the day's work. Activities such as music or dance are best if your work is more physical, otherwise you can run, walk fast or go to the gym.

If you wish to lose weight, exercise to increase your heart rate and raise a sweat. This more powerful exercise is required to burn excessive fat, but only to a level at which you feel comfortable and follow the rules of Yin and Yang balance. If your body is tired after too much work, you will lack energy.

In this case you need to rest, do gentle exercise, listen to or dance to relaxing music, or meditate. This will restore Yang energy to meet the body's needs, especially the metabolism, otherwise your body function will slow down, the mind will become exhausted and you will end up gaining more weight.

There are many ways to lose weight; activities other than exercise can help, but this works in a different way. I want also to emphasise the importance of sleep. Changing your sleep cycle or not getting enough sleep because of work or social commitments is fine occasionally, but getting enough sleep is very important in helping the body repair cells and detoxing. Lack of sleep is harmful, it can result in headaches, physical pain, or toxin overload.

YIN AND YANG IN FOOD

Traditional Chinese Medicine categorizes food according to four Qi and five flavours. The attributes of food and their relationship to Yin and Yang balance are well known to the Chinese – they are similar to the attributes of Chinese medicine. This knowledge guides people in which foods to eat and recipes to cook for wellbeing. For example, if you suffer from chronic stomach discomfort or an ulcer you should eat Chinese rice porridge every day – nothing else. After two days, your stomach should recover and your stomach ulcer should heal gradually over a few months.

The four Qi (四气) are: cool, hot, warm and cold. Cold and cool are Yin attributes, warm and hot are Yang attributes.

Cold and cool foods reduce the levels of Yang energy and increase Yin energy. It is beneficial to slow down the system and calm the mind, which will help relieve stress and skin irritation. If cold or cool food is eaten to excess or too often, it can damage Yang energy levels. This causes tiredness, slows the metabolism, and causes bloating, gas and a low mood.

Warm and hot foods increase the level of Yang energy and reduce Yin energy. It speeds up the body functions and mind. If warm or hot (spicy) food is eaten to excess or too often, the result is excessive heat in the body, causing anxiety and constipation. It also provides energy quickly. It will slow down the burning of fat, causing weight gain.

The five flavours (五味) of food are: sour (酸), sweet (甘), bitter (苦), spicy (辛) and salty (咸). Each flavour plays a different role in the body, affecting different internal organ functions.

Sour, sweet and spicy are Yang flavours and have an important role to play in wellbeing:

- Sour (vinegar taste) is a little sweet and a little bitter. It boosts Yang energy and Yin energy. It helps the liver to digest fatty food and kills bad bacteria and germs in the body system. Too much vinegar, however, causes stomach acid because Yin and Yang balance has been lost.
- Sweet is a Yang flavour. It relates to the spleen (which is linked to the metabolism). A small amount of sugar every day will boost Yang energy. People love sugar but too much sugar in the diet will slow down the body's energy system and metabolism. Also, sugar can quickly provide Yang energy as your body needs it. It will disturb the burning of fat in general and leads to weight gain.
- Spicy is a hot flavour, which relates to the lung, liver and spleen. It easily boosts Yang energy, but it also reduces your Yin energy. Eating too much

or too frequently causes excessive heat which increases the appetite, hunger, constipation and skin problems. This not only leads to weight gain, it can also cause other health issues.

- Salty and bitter are Yin flavours and also have an important role in body maintenance, detoxing, eliminating excessive heat, calming and relaxing.

- Salty flavours are a Yin energy and beneficial for muscle strength. Only a small amount is necessary. Too much salt can damage kidney function, leading to water retention, high blood pressure and weight gain.

- Bitter flavours are cold and Yin energy, which relates to the heart, lung and liver. It helps to calm the mind and reduce body heat. Eating a moderate amount is beneficial for skin problems. In excess, it can upset the digestive system which reduces Yang energy levels and slows the metabolism. The results in weight gain.

What I want to tell you is that, in principle, you can eat anything you like provided you do not eat too much of one food or too often. Otherwise, your body will lose Yin and Yang balance. This causes illness. As the Chinese say, 'an imbalance in food leads to an unhealthy body'.

The Table below sets out how certain foods of vegetables and sources can enhance Yin and Yang balance, and is a helpful guide on how certain foods affect your body, in both a positive and negative way:

THE YIN YANG GUIDE TO WEIGHT LOSS

Five Flavours	Four Chi	Yin/ Yang	Effect – Positive / Negative	Food
Sweet	Warm	Yang	Good Yang energy, calming effect on the stomach	pumpkin, honey, meat, seafood and fish, eggs, milk, potatoes, tomatoes
Salty	Cold/cool	Yin	Increases muscle strength in the kidneys, water retention in bladder	ham, bacon, mint tea, salt, salty meat
Sour	Warm/ hot	Yang	Anti-inflammatory for the liver and detoxification of the gall bladder	lemons, tomatoes oranges, olives, plums, vinegar
Bitter	Cold	Yin	Anti-inflammatory for the heart and detoxification of the small intestine	lettuce, green tea, asparagus mint tea
Spicy	Hot/ warm	Yang	Promotes circulation in the lungs but can cause constipation in the large intestine	ginger, onion, leeks, garlic, black pepper, chilli

Some foods may possess two or more different tastes, whereas some foods are relatively tasteless. For example:

Tomatoes are both sweet and sour. They are 'warm' and enhance your Yang energy, with a positive effect on the stomach, spleen, liver and gall bladder. They:

- Are easily digested, so helps the stomach
- Help the spleen, speed up the metabolism, and reduce body weight
- Help the liver, thus keeping you relaxed and stress-free
- Increase the production of citric acid and malic acid, thus helping the gall bladder function. The same is true of vinegar. (Modern research suggests vinegar can prevent kidney stones, fight inflammation and help with general detoxing)

Black pepper is spicy and warm, it enhances Yang energy and has a positive effect on the lung and large intestine:

- It helps increase lung Qi and is, particularly good if you suffer from chronic shortness of breath, fatigue, or swollen eyelids in the morning.
- It also helps to increase the Qi and Yang of the large intestine, which is particularly good if you suffer from bloating, wind, have cold hands or feet, or suffer from abdominal pain. It really helps to just add a little bit of black pepper into your meal.

Some foods are tasteless such as black mushroom, black fungus and tofu. They are all Yang energy food and as experience from history shows they are a replacement for animal fat in a vegetarian and vegan diet (discussed further in Chapter 6).

My recipes are always developed according to the attributes of the food to ensure good Yin and Yang balance. Food values in Yin and Yang are not absolute and they change. More information is provided in Chapter 7 – Guidelines for Recipes.

Food is heaven

There is an old Chinese saying: 'Food is heaven'. Food is a basic need and hunger breeds discontent. Food is one of the essentials of life, eating with family, friend and at celebrations is an enjoyment for us all.

The Chinese love cooking and eating. People who can cook delicious food are welcomed and respected in Chinese society. Knowledge is shared and people teach each other about cooking and diet – there are no formal lessons in ordinary families. But the Chinese have excellent recipes and a food culture that is deep in their history. Numerous recipes books have been passed down the generations. Everyone understands the attributes of food and the principles of Yin and Yang balance. This is the secret to why the Chinese stay slim.

I learned to cook when I was a teenager. My mother was a good, self-taught cook, who loved to teach me. I would watch her from a bench and I was always the first to test her food and tell her how good it tasted. Life was simple then compared to today. We had no TV, no mobile phones...not even a telephone. This was one of my enjoyments and it was fun to learn to cook.

Cooking is a crucial skill in Chinese life because it concerns the wellbeing of the person and plays a big part of family and social life. It is a common thing that we talk about doing every day. In China, meals play an important part of business dealings; they prefer to do business agreements around the dinner table rather than in the office.

Chinese people eat three times a day: breakfast, lunch and dinner in accordance with the body's natural cycle. Morning breakfast provides energy for the whole day, lunch provides energy for half the day, and the evening meal provides the minimum energy for the body to maintain its needs.

Each meal has a minimum of four different considerations: solid food (rices, noodles), soup, vegetables, and animal fat (fish, seafood or meat). If you are vegetarian or vegan use black mushrooms, black fungus or tofu etc. to replace animal fat. If somebody is sick, or recovering from childbirth or surgery, they should eat frequent but small portions.

Chinese people care about the quality of foods. More and more they prefer fresh, seasonal and organic food and are against vegetables or meat which are fast grown by chemicals in an artificial environment with additives to provide a longer shelf life. These unnatural elements are believed to be harmful to our wellbeing, believing organic is easier to digest and absorb less toxins.

The eating and cooking environment should be relaxed. Your digestion system works well if you are in a happy mood and not under stress. Eating is an enjoyment which helps to reduce stress levels.

Learning and practicing recipes is relaxing and interesting activity, a way to wellbeing without medication. Chinese people love and enjoy their food.

Hunger and weight loss

If you have suffered from weight gain, whether a lot or just a few pounds, you can lose weight by following the dietary principles, known as the 'hungry' method. It works within the framework of Yin and Yang balance. It is easily followed and can be done stress-free without disturbing your normal life.

The principle of this diet is that you should be 30% hungry after eating (achieving this gradually) There is an old Chinese saying, 'Stay one third hungry and cold, health is safe'. As Chinese people have experienced, your body only needs 70% of what you eat. This applies only to healthy people or those who are overweight. It does not apply to children, pregnant women or the sick.

Daily energy levels are driven by what we take in and what we excrete. There is a balance when you only consume what the body needs and therefore you will not gain weight. When you start cutting 10% to 30%

of your food intake as a gradual process, you will lose weight as a result. Normally this progress takes about a month to achieve, some people may take longer. Because you are cutting your food intake gradually without the body noticing you will feel normal with your new Yin and Yang balance level. This new balanced energy level will be sufficient for your needs. This is the central core to the Chinese remaining slim.

The reduction in food should be calculated based on the size of your regular daily meals. You should stop when you reach your desired body weight. This method of losing weight can also be used in conjunction with other methods of weight loss.

Controlling diet is important but it's vital to maintain Yin and Yang balance.

In 2009, I treated one patient very successfully with Chinese recipes and a change of lifestyle. He was 61 years old, overweight and had genetically high cholesterol. He would eat fish, vegetables, and up to a kilo of fruit every day. He believed he was following a healthy diet, yet he was frequently tired, had difficulty concentrating and suffered from bloating.

In his 20s, his father died suddenly of a heart attack at the age of 60, so he often visited his GP and took medicine for high cholesterol. But he was constantly struggling to lose weight. I gave him a long lesson in the Chinese philosophy of Yin and Yang balance, but he was initially sceptical about Chinese medicine. I decided to convince him about the benefits of the Chinese diet and Chinese lifestyle and suggested he alter his food consumption. He reduced his fruit intake from one or more kilograms a day to one apple, one banana and two pieces of melon. For breakfast, he would have hot milk, eggs with salmon or porridge; lunch and dinner would be salad with salmon, steamed sea bass, steamed vegetables or Chinese rice soup mixed with seafood, ginger and onion. After a period of time, he had improved energy levels and a slimmer physique.

Chinese people do not eat what they want, I told him. They eat in accordance with their body's needs whilst always striking a Yin and Yang balance.

CHAPTER 4

Differences in the Chinese and English Way of Living

There are many differences in the British (Western) food culture and life style compared to that of the Chinese. These differences result in difficulties for many in the West to stay slim and are the cause of many Western health problems too.

The key difference in the Chinese and British food culture and lifestyle lies in the Chinese philosophy of Yin and Yang balance. Let me explain what that means.

Yin and Yang governs the food you eat, when you eat, portion size and generally how you live your life. Living according to the principle of Yin and Yang balance is the secret behind the slim and healthy Chinese. To enjoy a healthy lifestyle, the body must enjoy Yin and Yang balance. Yin energy ensures body maintenance. Yang energy enhances activity.

The physical body, i.e. the organs, skin and bones, and

the functionand activities of the body represent Yang energy. The blood, bodily fluids and body tissues etc. represent the Yin energy.

The Chinese consider all food to have Yin and Yang attributes. Take the example of red meat. The Yin attributes of red meat enhance the blood levels while the Yang attributes improve the body's strength; Yin and Yang together help the growth of hair, skin, muscle and bone.

The Yin and Yang attributes of food differ according to the foods they are paired within colour, size, taste and attitude of the four Qi. For example:

- Green colour vs. red colour in food: green is Yin, red is Yang
- Light colour vs. dark colour in food: light is Yin, dark is Yang
- Meat vs. seafood: seafood is Yin, meat is Yang
- Meat vs. seafood vs. vegetables: meat and seafood are Yang, vegetables are Yin
- Tofu (soya beans) vs. vegetables: tofu is Yang, vegetables are Yin
- Solid food vs. liquid food (soup): solid food is Yang, liquid food (soup) is Yin
- Big portion vs. small portion: a big portion is Yang, a small portion is Yin

In the West, the energy value in food is measured in calories. Whether viewed from a Chinese or Western perspective, energy – be it Yin and Yang or calories – is gained and burned from diet, exercise and lifestyle.

Problems with Calories

The Western approach to weight loss and maintaining a healthy weight, is down to calorie consumption. Many of those who are dieting hope that by reducing their calorie consumption the body will react and achieve that dream drop in dress size. But do our bodies really function in such a simple way? The answer, sadly, is no.

In general, people understand that calories provide the human body with energy. To maintain a stable weight, the calories we put into our bodies must match the amount we need for daily living. If we consume more than we need, any excess will be stored as fat, leading to weight gain. But if we have too few calories in our diets, the body will function at a much slower pace and we will be tired. It's logical. If we can't function properly, the metabolism rate will slow down, causing water retention and an increase in toxins. Water retention and toxins lead to an increase in body weight. The quest to be slim will fail.

Some people can temporarily decrease their calorie intake to lose weight, but after a period this will no longer work. Many people complain that even though they eat very little calories they are still gaining weight. So what is going on?

The truth is that calorie control alone is not an effective way to lose weight. The most effective way of losing weight, and maintaining a healthy weight, is to master the philosophy of Yin and Yang balance in food and eat a balanced diet.

Here are a few examples of the problems I have encountered among those who are dieting:

- Eating only low-calorie food such as vegetables. Vegetables are a rich source of Yin energy but a poor source of Yang energy. Because there is a Yin and Yang imbalance in their diet, their energy deceases, bodily functions slow, then they feel tired and suffer from gas and bloating. To lose weight the metabolism must function well so that the body burns more fat, but the body needs the energy to achieve it. As a result, they are not getting sufficient calories to meet the body's needs for maintenance and activity. This can even cause weight gain.
- Skipping meals to reduce daily calorie intake hoping that the body will burn fat to provide the energy it needs to function. This approach will not succeed as the body burns fat at its own pace, the body system loses its normal routine, body function becomes poor and the result is weight gain.

In China, people eat according to what their body needs and choose foods to strike a Yin and Yang balance. If they want to lose weight, they will plan to:

- Cut the amount of food in their diet by a small percentage until they are satisfied with their weight. They will leave the table feeling 30%

hungry. Reducing food intake slowly to reach 30% will allow the body to properly adjust. It still retains Yin and Yang balance, i.e. if they normally have four dishes in one meal, they will still have four dishes, the ingredients will be the same, only the portion size will decrease.

- Select ingredients that are low in both Yin and Yang so that levels of Yin and Yang remain balanced. For example, if they frequently eat watermelon, which is sweet, they will replace it with cucumber.
- Drink Chinese tea if they are feeling hungry – not only does it help to ease hunger it is good for detoxing. Alternatively, if hungry, they will eat cucumber or white radish instead of fruits which contains lots of sugar.
- Exercise as often as your energy levels allow.

Remember, the body is not a one piece machine. Each part has different nutritional needs, which should not be switched off.

When Chinese families have dinner together, they have a lot of different ingredients in one meal. The meal will comprise of at least three to four dishes: soup, meat or seafood mixed with vegetables, and mixed vegetables. There will be different tastes, flavour and colour. The food will be delicious and easy to digest. They will eat lots of food happily and joyfully and they will remain slim.

I met Susan in March 2016. She worked twelve hour

days in IT in the City of London and was upset and stressed about her weight. Her best friend was getting married in May and she wanted to look her best for the wedding. She had been on a diet for two months, eating only fruit and vegetables and she exercised for up to an hour five times a week.

The problem was her weight was not dropping. In fact, she had actually gained some weight. She suffered from bloating, gas and constipation and her periods were delayed. What was the issue? There was not enough Yang energy food in her diet to fuel the long hours of work and frequent exercise, so her Qi energy was low. Her metabolism could not function properly, leading to water retention and weight gain.

The solution was to balance the number of calories spread between Yin and Yang foods, with a decent portion for each meal to match the needs of her activities. She started running every other day. Two weeks later, she was losing weight and eventually she managed to achieve her dream.

So, to summarise, the Chinese diet does not calculate calories; it follows the Yin and Yang balance.

Can we skip meals sometimes? My advice is that occasionally we can, but this is not a long term solution. Also remember that eating well is essential to happiness; irregular eating can result in bad moods and poor performance in the workplace.

Animal fat

Many people are scared of animal fat. Some health experts advise that animal fat should be eliminated from the diet to manage body weight. Some people believe body fat and animal fat are same thing. People are also confused about the relationship between animal fat and bad cholesterol. Lots of people have the impression that animal fat = bad cholesterol = body fat. But in fact, animal fat contains some good cholesterol which cannot be provided by any other food and is excellent for maintaining good health.

Does eliminating animal fat from your diet result in weight loss? The honest answer is no. Many people eat no animal fat but still have weight problems.

In Western medicine, fat is considered essential for body maintenance and function. It builds muscle, provides strength, protects organs and aids memory. Many nutrients including vitamins A, D, E and K are fat-soluble – the body cannot absorb them without fat. A fat-free diet can also lead to dry skin, brittle bones and muscle pains.

Clinical trials from the University of Minnesota Medical School suggest that: 'vitamin E is a powerful antioxidant and helps maintain our metabolism, while the body's level of vitamin D predicts its ability to lose fat, especially in the abdominal area'. Yes, it is true, 1 gram of fat has 9 calories – twice as many as carbohydrates or protein – but animal fat provides the best energy. It helps us to work and exercise, reduces problems with constipation and improves mood. Of course, eating more animal fat than the body needs will lead to weight gain, but other foods have the same effect. Even vegetables, if you eat more than your body needs, will cause you to gain weight.

Traditional Chinese medicine considers animal fat (from red meat, white meat or seafood) to be a very important Yang energy food. It is well known that the Chinese eat any kind of animal fat because they believe that it provides the best Yang energy and Qi energy. Yang and Qi energy are responsible for good body function generally, and specifically for the brain, the memory, strength in the heart cells and fertility organs.

In fact, animal fat has both Yang energy and Yin energy. The Yang improves the functioning of the kidneys, liver, spleen, heart and brain, etc. The Yin energy in animal fat enhances the whole body including the blood and bodily fluids it is maintaining. As a general rule, when people completely eliminate animal fat, they can suffer from low energy, a pale complexion, dry hair and skin, become moody and get stressed easily.

There is no evidence to show that people who have animal fat in their diet are less healthy than those who eat no animal fat.

In summary, it's an over-simplified judgements that animal fat equals body fat, which ignores the scientific information that animal fat provides our body with essential nutrition. Furthermore, animal fat and body fat behave completely differently in the body. Animal fat changes into nutrition as it goes through the body and has Yin and Yang balance. Body fat gained from over eating, bad eating habits or irregular meals lacks Yin and Yang balance. This lack of balance results in water retention and weight gain. To get the right solution to weight loss, it is crucial to understand how the human body works.

Problems Caused by Sugar

A significant difference in the diets of the British compared to the Chinese is the habit of drinking tea and coffee. In the West, people drink coffee and tea to boast energy while the Chinese drink tea for wellbeing and detoxing the body.

The British consume a lot of sugar with their coffee and tea, in additioin to cakes and desserts. I often joke with my family and friends, saying: 'English people are always so sweet because they eat so much sweet food'.

It is not unusual for the British to drink at least one or two cups of coffee every day. Often they will take it with sugar – 1 to 2 teaspoons per cup. Each teaspoon of sugar = 3 grams. A portion of dessert will probably have an additional 1-2 teaspoons of sugar. There is no doubt that heavy sugar consumption leads to weight gain and can lead to health problems.

My partner is English. When I first met him eight years ago he ate five times more sugar than me per day. Each day, he had 2-3 coffees with 2 teaspoons of sugar in each cup. He also loved cakes, sweets, and drank 1-2 glasses of wine per day. Personally, I don't add any extra sugar to my diet, only what occurs naturally in my food. I also don't drink coffee or wine. As a result, my partner was overweight while I was slim. But now that he has changed his diet and lifestyle, he has lost weight and got rid of some health issues.

The Chinese, in contrast, drink tea (without milk or sugar) that is a little bitter. They rarely drink coffee, or eat desserts and only eat naturally occurring plant sugar contained in vegetables and fruit, and in animal fat.

If you have a normal diet, you do not need extra sugar. Sugar provides the body with a quick source of Yang energy but the body doesn't need much: men need 9 teaspoons per day / women need 6 teaspoon per day.

In modern Western medicine, sugar is not considered to be necessary for the metabolism and humans do not produce it. In fact, it is mainly used by liver cells. When we eat a lot of sugar, most of the fructose is metabolised by the liver, where it turns into fat which is then secreted into the bloodstream for the whole body's system to use. Too much sugar results in a fatty liver. The excess is converted into fat for storage. Our *fat* cells are capable of creating chemical signals that lead to chronic inflammation caused by sugar. This inflammation can cause problems such as cancer, fatty liver, tumour, diabetes, etc. Because sugar is high in calories and can give the body energy more quickly than other foods, it disturbs the burning of fat and instantly stops weight loss.

Traditional Chinese Medicine regards sugar to be a source of Yang energy. Too much sugar slows the spleen function, which is related to the metabolism. When the spleen function slows, the metabolism rate slows. This causes constipation, bloating, tiredness and slowing of the memory. When the metabolism rate is slow, the body produces toxins which leads to water retention, weight gain and other health disorders.

Refined sugar is not eaten in China, nor are chemically based sweeteners. The body's daily sugar needs are gained from fruit, vegetables and some meats. Plant sugar is natural, healthy and it does not change the body's signalling system. As a result, it does not disturb normal body function. Used long term, refined sugar and chemically based sweeteners will change the body signalling system and cause changes to the body system.

Traditional Chinese medicine and Western medicine are united in their advice on sugar – it is bad for your health. For good health and wellbeing, and for weight loss, sugar should be eliminated from your diet as much as you can.

A love of potatoes

The British have the same fondness for potatoes as the Chinese have for rice. The love affair with potatoes could have something to do with the climate as potatoes easily fill you up and quell hunger in cold conditions.

In China, the potato is regarded as one of many vegetables. People tend to eat potatoes once or twice a week when they are in season. We are often amazed by the variety of ways in which the English eat potatoes, e.g. chips, roast potatoes, mashed potatoes, baked potatoes, etc. – they appear to eat potatoes all the time. Fish and chip shops are a source of puzzlement to the Chinese – they sell only two food types, fish and chips, and there are many of them!

The Chinese cannot live without rice and it seems the British cannot live without potatoes.

Potatoes can be tasty and delicious – but they can also cause weight problems and, in excess, are not good for wellbeing as they slow the metabolism. Big portions of potatoes fill you up leaving little room for other vegetables. If someone eats potato as the main part of their diet, they may suffer from bloating, gas, low energy, and weight gain.

As I have emphasised many times, healthy eating and living requires a diet based on the principles of Yin and Yang balance. Different foods have different energy sources – when you regularly eat too much potato, the body gradually loses Yin and Yang balance.

I have on occasion recommended to my clients that they should eat rice. Some of them told me they found it easy on their digestive system. In Traditional Chinese Medicine books written two thousand years ago, Chinese rich porridge was used as a herbal prescription to treat digestive disorders and as a cure for colds, flus and morning sickness. It is still highly recommended today as a simple medicine to patients suffering from cancer, liver problems or when recovering from surgery.

Cheese and Butter

I conducted some research on the impact of cheese, butter and sunflower oil on health, and the findings shocked me. The table below lists how much fat, cholesterol and sodium is contained in 100g.

	Sunflower Oil	Cheese	Butter
Fat	100g	33g	81g
Saturated Fat	0	21g	51g
Cholesterol	0	105mg	215mg
Sodium	0	621mg	11mg

You probably know that saturated fat does not have a good reputation in modern Western medicine. This is because saturated fat is believed to increase the levels of cholesterol in the blood. In turn, this can increase the risk of heart disease and heart attacks. It can also cause narrowing of the arteries (atherosclerosis) and weight gain.

Cholesterol is a fatty substance made by your liver and carried around the body in the blood. Fats in food you eat can affect the levels of cholesterol in your blood.

There is a lot of sodium in cheese, which is a major cause of water retention and weight gain. There is no cheese or butter in the Chinese diet, but in England they both feature frequently in meals and fill large sections of the supermarkets.

Cheese and butter are the animal products most detrimental to good health in the Western diet. In addition, they cause weight gain. Give up this unhealthy food and your health will be better.

Alcohol

The British people's love for alcohol goes back many centuries and pubs are popular social spaces. In a 17th century diary entry, Samuel Pepys described the pub as 'the heart of England'.

Beer, wine and spirits are drunk at all kinds of gatherings with friends. And having a drink after work is part of the daily routine for many people. When English people visit friends the first thing they do is offer them a drink. They drink when they are happy, sad or stressed.

One or two normal sized glasses of wine per night is fine, it is enjoyable, good for relaxation and good for blood circulation to the heart and joints. However, the benefit is lost if you drink to excess – it is bad for your health.

Wine and spirits are high in sugar and alcohol – both are detrimental to slimming. We know that the body requires very little sugar; its needs can be supplied by the fruit and vegetables eaten as part of a normal diet. Sugar is the enemy of weight loss.

Alcohol too can be detrimental to weight loss and wellbeing. Normally, the liver metabolises fat calories allowing them to be used for energy. When you drink alcohol, the breakdown of fat becomes secondary to the breakdown of alcohol. Instead of using fat for energy, your body turns to the calories from the alcohol. This causes a build-up of fatty acids that can hinder weight loss. In addition, alcohol increases your appetite, makes you hungry, causing you to eat more. Alcohol also makes you thirsty, causing you to drink more water than your body may need. This causes weight gain.

Taken to excess over time, alcohol can change the body's signalling system. This can lead to: difficulty in switching off the mind, lack of focus, heart problems and alcohol addiction. It can also lead to changes in the physical body, which can cause cancer, diabetes and heart problems.

Chinese wine is made from rice. It is high in alcohol but very low in sugar. The Chinese drink wine at meal times and then only on special occasions such as celebrations, parties, business meetings or dinners.

By comparison, the British do not necessarily see wine as a drink that goes with food. It can be drunk at virtually any time of the day.

Wine is a source of Yang energy. Too much Yang energy results in an imbalance between Yin and Yang energy and causes the fluid circulation of the body to speed up. When wine is consumed with food, the body is likely to maintain the Yin and Yang balance.

Junk Food and Processed Meals

Tesco was forced to withdraw from the Chinese market because it failed to understand the local food culture.The Chinese do not like fast food or prepared dishes. They prefer fresh and organic produce. Organic food is natural and shares the same root with the human body – they form part of the natural order. Organic food enhances body maintenance and the body's ability to undertake physical activity.

Some English people have lost interest in cooking at home – particularly the younger generation.

Why should we cook food at home? The answer is simple: home-cooked food is fresh, organic and provides a greater choice for the body. Choose between different vegetables, meat, or mixed seafood to satisfy your body's needs. When you cook food, you can design your own recipes according to taste. Cooked food is easier to digest and requires less energy from the body.

All that additional energy can be invested in other activities. Home-cooked food can also be shared with friends and family, improving your social life. It tastes better, lasts longer, and produces less toxins in your body. Choose the correct Yin and Yang balance of recipes and you will notice an improvement in health.

We know that junk food and processed meals cause weight gain and are bad for your health. Why is this?

Firstly, junk food contains very high levels of salt and sugar, artificial flavour and chemical preservatives. Salt and chemical preservatives prolong the shelf life of junk food while artificial flavour and added sugar make it taste good.

Too much salt and sugar cause weight gain and are harmful to the body, as are chemical preservatives. Junk food is not natural and can also contain genetically modified ingredients. Independent studies have linked genetically modified food to birth defects, organ failure, infertility and cancers.

Secondly, junk food does not contain sufficient levels of essential vitamins and minerals and is high in calories.

This lack of essential vitamins and minerals will, in the longer term, damage body maintenance and lead to poor body function. High calories cause the body to burn less fat and cause weight gain.

Thirdly, the synthetic ingredients in junk food can harm the body by interfering with the metabolism and changing the internal body environment. Those problems can lead to weight gain and cause fatigue, acidosis and other health problems.

Many Chinese and Western health experts are opposed to junk food and processed meals. Protecting our generations health is important. We must take action now and eliminate junk food from our diet.

Family life

Culturally, English people value individualism and are very independent and self-sufficient. The Chinese, on the other hand, are more family oriented; they talk to each other, support each other, make dinner together and share their feelings more. Having a strong support network can reduce stress, which is a major contributor to weight gain.

The Chinese family lifestyle has two main health benefits:

- Sharing a family meal together promotes knowledge of food and nutrition, helps refine cooking skills, encourages for experimentation with recipes, and brings enjoyment. On top of that seasonal, organic food cooked at home is much more nourishing than restaurant cooked food.

- Taking a family meal together helps family members reduce stress from the day's work and other social pressures. Stress is the root cause of many serious health problems, including weight gain.

To conclude, the British and the Chinese have very different philosophies, cultures and customs when it comes to food. This chapter provides the detailed explanations on how Chinese people achieve slim figures and wellbeing effortlessly through their eating habits.

CHAPTER 5

Common Mistakes
to Make
in Weight Loss

I have found that many people fail in their efforts to lose weight. This may be because there is a misunderstanding about what dieting involves. There is a common misconception about the role of lifestyle in dieting and weight loss or people do not understand why they gain weight in the first place.

Here I have listed some of the common problems faced by slimmers. Based on my own experience I will explain through the medium of case-studies how and why slimmers make these common mistakes and I will outline the best way to lose weight.

WHY CAN'T I LOSE WEIGHT ON A VEGETARIAN DIET?

There are nearly four million vegetarians in the UK – some for religious reasons, others want to avoid cruelty to animals. More and more, however, vegetarianism has become more popular due to various health problems which have arisen that are related to diet and lifestyle. People think that rejecting a normal diet in favour of becoming vegetarian will help with these issues of wellbeing and weight loss.

Some people think their diet has caused their weight gain and that being vegetarian helps with weight loss. There are also individuals who have followed a vegetarian diet but have failed to lose weight. In these cases, it is necessary to establish the underlying reasons for the weight gain.

Here I will discuss on a case by case basis weight gain due to diet. It should be remembered that there are many reasons for weight gain including hormones, stress, liver and kidney problems, etc.

In Chinese philosophy, provided your diet has Yin and Yang balance, you will not gain weight. To lose weight you should cut the portion size at each meal, starting with the evening meal, and ensuring that Yin and Yang balance is maintained. To succeed, you also need to ensure that you are eating enough to meet your body's minimum physical activity and maintenance need.

Changing your diet from normal to vegetarian, eating the same food with the exclusion of animal products, is unlikely to help you to lose weight. You will be successful in losing weight if you adopt the principles of Yin and Yang balance, regardless of whether your diet is normal, vegetarian or vegan.

Let me tell you the story of my retired London friends, Victoria and David. David lost four friends and a classmate to cancer and heart problems in a six month period. Shocked by this, they started to worry about their own health and diet. David enjoys a drink, is slim and fit and has a non-red meat diet. Victoria has a normal diet, health and average weight.

They decided to adopt a vegan diet. A year later, Victoria was admitted to A&E suffering from a severe deficiency of haemoglobin and iron. She was weak, tired and suffering from water retention. The doctor advised an immediate blood transfusion and iron pills, which she refused. David was also suffering froma fatty liver and massive weight gain. They sought my advise urgently. I prescribed the following for both of them:

1) A Yin and Yang balanced diet to include red meat, vegetables and tofu, which is rich in iron and energy
2) Daily exercise or other physical activities, taken outdoor in the sun and fresh air.
3) Keeping stress to a minimum

The purpose was to reduce water retention, help with weight loss and regain liver function. Two months later, Victoria's haemoglobin and iron levels were back to normal and David had regained his energy and lost weight. Today they are fit, slim and healthy.

The conclusion was that their vegan diet had been unbalanced.

Still I hear people say that a vegan or vegetation diet can keep them slim. They cite as evidence the fact that Chinese

Taoism and Buddhism support non-meat diets and they enjoy a long life. The truth is Taoists and Buddhists are vegetarian for religious reasons and not because a vegetarian diet is healthier than a normal diet. They also undertake lots of physical activity every day out in the sun and fresh air, and eat seasonal organic food in accordance with the principles of Yin and Yang balance. It is the totality of this lifestyle which keeps them fit and healthy.

The table below compares the differences between the typical Western, Buddhist and Taoist ways of life. It demonstrates that their diet and lifestyle have nothing in common with a Western diet and lifestyle.

People	Taoism	Buddhism	English
Food Supply	Organic	Organic	Organic or Non-organic
Drink	Chinese Tea, Water	Chinese Tea, Water	English tea, Coffee, Wine, Beer
Exercise	2-3 hours per day Martial arts, Climbing, Walking	2-3 hours per day Martial arts, Climbing, Walking	Gym 30 minutes to 1 hour, 2-3 times a week or none
Daily Transport	Walk	Walk	Bus, Tube, Car
Work	Study	Study	Sitting at

	Physical work out doors	Physical work out doors	computer or physical work indoors
Stress Score	+	+	++++
TV or mobile phone	None	None	2-3 hours minimum
Workplace	Mountain	Mountain	City Office
Time spent outdoors	6-8 hours every day except in bad weather	6-8 hours every day except in bad weather	Less than 1-2 hours per day

Conclusion: In the West, people who want to be slim think in terms of calories, fat and exercise. In China, people look at all aspects of life; they think holistically in terms of lifestyle, stress, hours of work, leisure time, living environment and happiness. There is a philosophical difference in approach.

WHY CAN'T I LOSE WEIGHT WHEN I'M STRESSED?

Stress is an emotional response by the body to problems experienced at work and life, unrealised personal ambitions, relationship difficulties and other pressures. It can manifest as anxiety, depression, difficulty sleeping or over-eating, among others. Stress is also the enemy of weight loss. Traditional Chinese Medicine believes that stress effects a person's liver function.

Let me explain how the liver function is effected by stress and why it results in weight gain.

Traditional Chinese Medicine considers the liver as the manager of our emotions (肝主疏泄). Liver function is easily disturbed by excessive emotions or below normal emotions. When liver motions become excessive, you can easily become anxious, angry or excited. This is called Excessive Liver Yang (肝阳上亢). When liver motion levels are reduced, you will find yourself depressed, upset, with no interest in normal activates. This is called Liver Qi Stagnant.

- When the liver is stressed, it will affect other organ function, resulting in hunger or less activity and loss of appetite; constipation, or irregular bowel movement; sleeplessness, bloating and gas, water retention, etc.

The liver is in charge of cleaning and detoxing. A stressed liver causes Qi to become stagnant and stagnation of the blood (气滞血瘀). If the energy channel is blocked, body toxins are not removed in a timely manner – the toxins are not eliminated until the liver is able to resume its task.

- When blockage happens, it causes pain in the neck, shoulders or back; or the body changes these toxins to fat resulting in weight gain, or low energy etc.

I have one patient who gained weight due to serious stress suffered over the course of a year. Susan visited me in May 2017. She wanted to lose twenty pounds which she had gained following the break-up with her partner in April 2016.

She works as a financial consultant in the City of London. She was eating normally with no junk food or alcohol, and went to the gym three times a week. She sometimes felt tired, suffered from constipation and occasional gas, poor concentration and sleeplessness. Her periods had been irregular for eight months. I could see no reason other than stress for her condition and weight gain.

Her treatment plan was as follows:

- I explained the philosophy of Yin and Yang balance and prescribed a diet based on these principles with food chosen especially to nourish her body and help her liver detox.
- I advised her on what liquids to drink each day and gave her an exercise routine to help relieve her stress.

Diet: In the morning she should eat a normal breakfast sometimes interspersed with Chinese rice porridge as it is very good for the digestion and is a source of Yang energy. At lunch she should cut portion size but otherwise eat a normal meal to include warm soup and dishes based on tofu and meat. She should eat with colleagues to help alleviate stress and have a 5-10 minute nap. Her evening meal should be as usual, but she should avoid salad and include vegetable soup and cooked vegetables.

Liquid to detox her body: She should drink warm water, lemon tea or green tea throughout the day. Before bed, she should have a cup of warm water with a teaspoon of honey. This was to calm her and help with sleep and detoxing.

Exercise and physical activity: I prescribed a mixed programme of activities – on different days she should walk, run, join a group(s) where she could dance and on other days sing. To help keep her mind happy and relaxed, I also advised her to take part in other activities she found interesting, e.g., join a book club, go to the theatre and spend time with family and friends.

Additionally she had several sessions of slimming acupuncture, lymphatic massage, and cupping. She felt better after the first session, her body weight started to reduce from the first week. Once she had achieved her weight loss goals, she went on to live according to the principles of Yin and Yang balance.

WHY SHOULDN'T I DRINK TOO MUCH WATER WHEN TRYING TO LOSE WEIGHT?

Whether or not you are trying to lose weight, too much water is not good for you. Everybody needs a certain amount of water to maintain our body's needs, including replacing daily water loss and detoxing. Water is required by all the body's organs and systems – without it we would die.

In 2010, a report from The European Food Safety Authority suggested that the minimum levels of water consumption should be 10 glasses per day for men, 8 glasses per day for women. Included in this was the water gained from our daily intake of food, fruit and tea. Against this should be balanced levels of activity, state of health, your size, weight and whether the climate is hot or cold.

The Chinese have a different approach to the amount of water they drink daily. The amount they drink depends on: whether they feel thirsty, whether their skin or eyes are dry, whether or not they are constipated, or their joints are stiff. They will balance their daily intake against these physical signals from the body as to whether it has sufficient water or not.

Water in Traditional Chinese Medicine is a source of Yin energy and food is a Yang energy source. The amount eaten and drunk each day should be governed by the principles of Yin and Yang balance.

Traditional Chinese Medicine believes water is life-giving and crucial for good body balance. It particularly effects the functioning of the spleen (脾主运化) and the kidneys. Part of the spleen function equals the role of the metabolism in Western medicine, whilst the role of the kidney （肾主水） is similar to its role in Western medicine – to flush toxins from the liver and kidneys.

Let me explain the role drinking too much water plays in weight gain. In Traditional Chinese Medicine, the role of the spleen function (脾为后天之本) is to convert the intake of food and drink into energy (Yin and Yang) for body maintenance and activities. It also produces toxins in the form of waste and toxin water.

When you drink too much water, you will automatically eat less food. Whenyou are eating less food you will have less Yang energy, leading to a Yin and Yang imbalance. This can result in weight gain in several ways, such as;

- Excessive body water
- Body function slowing down; natural detoxing system becoming less effective; body toxins can change into fat
- Low energy resulting in the body burning less fat than normal

I recall one case of a patient whose failure to lose weight as a result of drinking too much water left a deep impression on me. Susan visited me in May 2016. She had been trying to lose weight for over two years, suffered from water retention, and chronic tiredness, had absent or delayed periods, was stressed due to being overweight and suffered from bloating and gas. She believed her diet was fairly normal.

I did not consider her diet to be in Yin and Yang balance. She was not eating sufficient at each meal to support her work, activities and maintenance of her body. She did not drink soft drinks or eat junk food and her exercise levels were normal. It was clear her very significant weight gain was not as a result of her diet. However, she was drinking massive amounts of water – up to six litres a day and sometimes eight. She was doing this because she believed water was good for her health, detoxing and weight loss. The truth was it was the cause of her weight gain.

Her treatment plan was as follows:

- I advised her on the philosophy of Yin and Yang balance and explained that the amount of water she was consuming could lead to liver and kidney failure.
- Gradually over a six week period cut down the amount of cold water she was drinking from 6 litres to 1.5 litres. The cold water was replaced by warm water, hot water with lemon or wu-long tea.
- Replace cold salads with steamed vegetables and exclude cold foods for the moment.
- Eat Chinese rice porridge for breakfast, vegetables or meat with vegetables, and vegetable soup for lunch and dinner. Because she was chronically tired, I increased the amount of Yang food (meat) in those meals but still ensured her diet was in Yin and Yang balance.
- Exercise or other activities to be taken outdoors to benefit from the fresh air and the sun, which also increases Yang energy. She should not exercise if she lacked the energy or was too tired. More strenuous exercise be mixed with relaxing, less demanding activities.

- After 6 weeks, she should drink warm water and tea as she felt like it rather than taking a prescribed amount – as the Chinese do.
- I prescribed some treatment to re-balance her body function.

She lost 8 kilos in 6 weeks, felt better and looked better. Now she is fit, slim and happy.

Science tells us that the female body is comprised of 55% water, the male body 65% water. The body needs water to allow the lungs and skin to breath, for urine and bowel activity, and to accommodate physical activity and the climate (hot or cold). We can replenish the body's water requirements by drinking water, tea, soup, and eating food, vegetables and fruit containing water. As a general rule you should drink six to eight glasses of water per day. If you do not feel thirsty, that is enough.

WHY CAN'T I LOSE WEIGHT BY DRINKING DIET DRINKS?

Diet drinks are not a natural source, they cannot play a role in your Yin and Yang balance.

Confusion surrounds the consumption of diet drinks. Factory produced, and containing refined sugar or artificial sweeteners and chemicals, they can be addictive, harmful to the body and are not a natural substance. Some scientific studies show no conclusive harmful effects to humans. Other studies link these sugar substitutes to cancers, tumours, and – ironically – weight gain.

Studies looking at large groups of people have shown obese people tend to drink more fizzy diet drinks than other people. In fact, a review by Imperial College London has argued that there is 'no solid evidence' that low-calorie sweeteners are any better for weight-loss than full sugar drinks.

Artificial sweeteners and refined sugar can change the body's natural ability to calculate its calorie needs and cause you to eat more. A study from Purdue University's Digestive Behavior Research Centre showed that rats given 'no calorie' sweeteners actually ate more thereby gaining more weight and body fat than rats that ate regular table sugar.

'Diet' does not mean calorie free, it means less calories. I have seen in my Weight Management Practice that people who regularly consume diet drinks over a long period lack energy, feel tired, their brain function slows, they lack concentration, suffer from poor memory and gain weight.

There is not yet any scientific evidence showing how consuming diet drinks causes weight gain as well as serious health problems. It is a fact however that since refined sugar, sweeteners and chemical additives have been widely used in the food industry, people are experiencing more and more health problems such as cancer, tumours and diabetes.

What do the Chinese think of diet drinks? The

Chinese believe natural food is good for the body – they prefer fresh food which should ideally be organic, or as near to organic as possible. Diet drinks contain: refined sugar, artificial sweeteners and chemicals, which effect the body as follows:

- They are not natural. When you consume diet drinks, your body does not recognise what it is being given and reacts as though it is being invaded by an enemy, e.g. a virus, an unknown bacteria or physical injuries. The body's defence system reacts gradually, such as low energy swelling, headaches, constipation, gas, bloating and fatty liver. In Western medicine the defence system consists of white cells or the lymphatic system. In Traditional Chinese Medicine, the defence system includes the liver, kidneys, and bladder.

- Refined sugar, artificial sweeteners and chemical additives can perhaps change the body system's natural environment. It can lead to gradual changes in the way the body normally functions, which may account for the increase in cancers and tumours since the introduction of these products into our diets. There is still no scientific evidence to confirm this but there is no doubt that people who consume these products on a long term basis suffer from weight gain and ill-health.

- Diet drinks are liquid food and a Yin energy source. If you drink them too much you will need less food. It will create a Yin and Yang inbalance leading to weight gain.

Steven visited me in 2015. He had gained weight since retiring three years earlier and could not understand why. He was not stressed, ate regular meals, played golf two or three times a week, was a member of a book club, did charity work and holidayed regularly with family and friends. However, he was addicted to diet drinks, consuming as many as four to five 250ml bottles every day. It was clear to me that the diet drinks were the cause of his weight gain but he had already tried and failed to stop.

I treated him by:

- Explaining the Chinese philosophy of Yin and Yang balance
- Advising him to immediately eliminate the diet drinks. I supported him with acupuncture and cupping to help with the symptoms caused by stopping, which included: anxiety, thirst, a funny taste in the mouth, stomach and nasal discomfort.

I continued this treatment combined with advise on living in accordance with the principles of Yin and Yang balance until he lost the excess weight. He has remained slim and enjoys his life.

If you have a similar habit of consuming diet drinks, you should take similar action and eliminate them from your diet.

WHY CAN'T I LOSE WEIGHT THROUGH USING NUTRITIONAL OR DIETARY SUPPLEMENTS?

Replacing food with nutritional or dietary supplements when trying to lose weight is not unusual. Nutritionists, dietitians and the health food industry often recommend their use in weight management programmes. There are many reasons for weight gain. Before trying to lose weight, it is important to understand the reason for your weight gain so that the underlying reason is correctly addressed. Taking nutritional or dietary supplements may not be the appropriate solution for you until you understand the reason for your weight gain.

The providers of these products believe that they can effectively replace carbohydrates or calories in the diet. It is true that you can control calories but these products never replace the foods needed to restore your body's natuaral balance.

It must be remembered that the body system, particularly the stomach, needs food regularly to feel full, the mouth requires natural tasting food and the digestive system needs to do its normal job of processing the food we eat. If these functions are disrupted their natural function will be lost over time. There is an old saying 'food is happiness'. An empty stomach on an ongoing basis can cause damage such as ulcers, gastritis and absent or irregular periods. These side effects are often down played.

Your body has its own routines, rather like that of

plants growing in the earth. Plants can live in artificial water or artificial earth, but it is not same as plants growing in their natural environment, the earth. Natural food is not the same as processed products and your body recognises this.

I have a patient who has taken dietary supplements for one year. She is over 50 years of age, a housewife who has never worked outside the home. She gained weight over a three year period following the menopause and had followed various slimming programmes, all of which had failed. Latterly, she had started taking dietary supplements on the advice of a neighbour.

She did lose weight dramatically during the first six months of taking the supplements but soon went on to suffer from stomach discomfort including severe acid reflux, sleeplessness, poor appetite and low energy. Hospital investigations found she had a stomach ulcer and gastritis. She decided to try alternative medicine rather than Western medicine and came to me for a consultation.

Her treatment plan was as follows:

- I educated her in the philosophy of Yin and Yang balance in health and lifestyle.
- I treated her ulcer, gastritis and tiredness with acupuncture, moxibustion and herbal tea.
- She stopped the dietary supplements and she resumed eating normal food after my consultation. I taught her how to select food to maintain Yin and Yang balance, and about fluid

intake to help her get more Yang energy and to detox.

- She had Chinese rice porridge in the morning and drank warm water or hot water with lemon. Lunch and evening meals consisted of soup and balanced Yin and Yang food. All the food she consumed was easy to digest and she avoided cold salads and cold food, hard nuts, yoghurt and wheat. Portion size was small and she commenced eating five meals a day, gradually decreasing to three, to allow the stomach to heal.

- Engaging in activities outside the home, including exercise in the sun and fresh air to enhance her hormonal balance and heal the body's injured Yin and Yang balance.

In the end, she was returned to good health and has remained fit and slim. She has continued to follow the Chinese diet and lifestyle.

WHY DOES EXERCISE NOT HELP ME LOSE WEIGHT?

Exercise is one of the most important physical activities for helping with weight loss and maintaining a good life balance. Exercise helps detoxify the body by eliminating waste and water in the breath and through the skin. After exercise, your mood is enhanced, the body feels lighter and the brain is refreshed.

I have been asked 'why is it that I have not lost weight when I eat a well-balanced diet and exercise regularly?' or people say 'I often exercise, but my energy is sometimes low and I am putting on weight'. Weight gain has many reasons, and you need to find your real root cause. You should not simply use exercise without correcting the problems that you suffer from, especially if you have been tired due to physical work causing low Yang energy. In the meantime, reducing your excessive exercise will result in more Yang energy, causing a Yin and Yang imbalance. It is not surprising that you will gain weight.

I will tell you about one of my patients who I met in July 2017 and maybe you will find the answer to your question...

Neil is a trader in the City. He needs a lot of energy to do his job. He is not overweight, but wished to lose a few pounds. He started going to the gym five times a week and cycled at the weekend. After two months, rather than losing weight he had gained a little. He worked twelve hour days, leaving his flat at 6.00 am and returning at 6.00 pm. He then went to the gym for 60-90 minutes where his workout included heavy lifting and running. He worked out until he was extremely tired. In the beginning he was OK with this routine but after about two weeks he began to feel more tired than before. He had to force himself to go to the gym because of lack of energy and exhaustion. He thought his tiredness was due to the long hours he worked. He continued to exercise as he considered he needed exercise to balance his long working day.

Of course, keeping a balance between work and exercise is right, but there was a lack of Yin and Yang balance in his approach. Because he worked very long hours, and spent the day sitting down, he was losing Yang energy. Added to this, his exercise programme was too powerful and too frequent, which further depleted his Yang energy.

The solution was for him to try and cut his hours of work if he could and to undertake a mixed programme of exercise. This included half of his exercise time spent walking, cycling in the park or countryside, doing tai chi or dancing, the other half working out in the gym to include running and heavy lifting. This programme returned his body to Yin and Yang balance, improved his energy levels and enabled him to lose weight.

He followed this programme and I taught him the principles of Yin and Yang balance. He lost the additional pounds in a short time and became fascinated with the philosophy of Yin and Yang balance to the extent that he is planning to go to China to do a philosophy course in Xi'an. A happy outcome!

I EAT FRUIT, NO ANIMAL FAT AND WHEAT, BUT I STILL KEEP GAINING WEIGHT. WHY?

People often ask me, 'why, if I eat lots of fruits, no animal fat and wheat, do I still keep gaining weight?'. My answer is that there is still problems with their Yin and Yang balance.

Meals need to be Yin and Yang balanced including your fruit and drink intake over a 24 hour cycle. It is easy to take the wrong action and find the outcome disappointing.

Commonly, fruits contain high sugar levels and a high percentage of water compared to vegetables. These two points can lead to weight problems.

If your body's daily sugar level increases more than your body needs, sugar will easily turn to fat and can also damage the liver. Sugar also quickly provides energy, so your body naturally reduces the fat it burns to provide that energy.

If your body has more water than it needs your body's original Yin and Yang balance will be disrupted. As you know, water is a Yin energy source and when your body's Yin energy increases your body function will slow down. In the West, they have the same option that excessive sugar and water can lead to body weight gain.

I met Ms Ann in 2016. She was over 65 years, retired for two years, and she had gained 5 kilos during this time. She had been on a weight loss programme for 3 months, went to the gym 3 times a week, ate less and had replaced 50% of her food intake of meat, rice and wheat with fruit. In the end, she ended up gaining a further kilo in this period. Additionally, she suffered from bloating and gas, and became tired easily. She did not have stress, in fact, she had lots of holidays and a normal 24-your routine I couldn't find any other issue for her body weight than her high fruit intake.

Her treatment plan was as follows:

- I educated her in the philosophy Yin and Yang balance in health and lifestyle.
- She resumed her normal diet, instead reducing her portion size by 5- 10%
- All food and drink needed to be in Yin and Yang balance. After two weeks, she no longer felt tired, bloated or had gas. She then started to reduce her meals by a further 5% . She practiced the Yin and Yang balance in food and lifestyle and succeeded in achieving her desired body size and feeling of wellbeing.

CHAPTER 6

Popular Teas, Fruits and Vegetables

Teas

China is one of the most important tea-producing countries. Its history extends as far back as 3,000 years ago, the same length of time as the history of Traditional Chinese medicine. In ancient China, tea was originally used as a medicine; over hundreds of years it slowly shifted towards being viewed first as a tonic and for detoxing, and then as a beverage as it is today.

Chinese people drink tea on average 3-4 times a day. Tea has many benefits, it enhances Yang energy and helps the body to function, aiding relaxation, helping digestion and detoxifying. It also enhances Yin energy, helps the body to repair, clears toxins and nourishes the skin.

Different teas have different functions according to its nutritional values in Yin and Yang energy. For example, green tea mainly helps the body to stay calm and is easily an aid to digestion whereas Wu-long tea helps the body to absorb oily or fatty food. Green tea, wu-long tea and camomile tea have the lowest calories making them ideal for everyday drinking.

Mint tea has high levels of: iron 28%, calcium 24%, vitamin A 85% and vitamin C 50% – excellent news for people suffering from deficiencies. In Chinese nutritional values, it calms the body's system and improves skin

Nowadays, it's possible to buy tea from all over the world. Sometimes it is difficult to choose the right tea, but always follow the Yin and Yang philosophy. Here are several ways to identify the Yin and Yang nutritional values:

- According to its attitude of five taste and four Qi: wu-long tea is warm, which is Yang; green tea is little cool, which is Yin. Ginger tea is spicy, which is yang; lemon tea is a litter bitter, which is Yin.
- According to colour: wu-long tea is brownish and dark-ish which is Yang; green tea is greenish, which is Yin.
- According to texture: camomile is soft, which is Yin; mint tea is hard, which is Yang.

Each tea's nutritional value depends on the ingredient, the climate and environmental factors such as sun, air, pollution and dryness etc. If tea is grown in strong sun with four very different seasons, fresh air and free of pollution, this tea will have more nutritional value than others.

Below I will state the nutritional information in the Chinese values of Yin and Yang, the nutricional benefits for the organs, and their nutritional values of calories, sugar, iron and vitamin C in a percentage value based on a 2000 calorie daily diet.

GREEN TEA

You can drink 2-3 cups every day but it is better not to drink after 6pm as it may disrupt sleep.
If you want green tea to counteract alcohol or oily/ fatty food that is bad for the liver, you can drink it immediately after.

Green tea grows in regions which have a warm, humid climate with a rainfall measuring at least 100 cm a year. Ideally, it likes deep, light, acidic and well-drained soil. The best tea will grow in areas from sea level up to altitudes as high as 2,100 metres above sea level on the higher mountains.

In Traditional Chinese medicine

Green tea is a great Yin and Yang energy source. It is sweet and a little bitter so it is beneficial to the liver, spleen, lungs and kidneys.

- It can improve Yang (Qi) energy, helping the body to function. It helps the spleen with Yang energy, speeding up digestive progress, reducing bloating and gas, and helping to reduce constipation. It helps the kidneys produce Yang energy by eradicating waste or unwanted water and reducing water retention.

- It can improve Yin energy, helping to maintain health. It boosts the liver in Yin energy, reducing stress, depression, anxiety, and helping to calm a busy mind. For helping the kidneys with Yin energy, it strengthens joints and reduces pain, and also helps the body to detox and cleanse.
- It can help fatty food and alcohol minimise toxins produced and remove toxins fast.
- It also regulates free Qi movement, reducing headaches, and neck and shoulder pain.

When you drink more green tea, in the long term your system will be healthier.

As stated, some of the health benefits of green tea are as follows:

- Helping the digestion system
- Helping weight loss
- Helping anti-ageing
- Helping the body system to detox
- Helps relaxation

One study from the University of Maryland Medical Centre (www.umin.com) found that: 'Green tea is made from unfermented leaves and reportedly contains the highest concentration of powerful antioxidants called polyphenols. Antioxidants are substances that fight free radicals, damaging compounds in the body that change cells, damage DNA, and even cause cell death. Many scientists believe that free radicals contribute to the aging process, as well as the development of a number of health problems, including cancer and heart disease.'

Antioxidants, such as polyphenols in green tea, can neutralise free radicals and may reduce or even help prevent some of the damage they cause.

Another article on the benefits of green tea (www.ncbi.nlm.gov.com) said: 'Long-term consumption of tea catechins could be beneficial against high-fat diet-induced obesity and type II diabetes, and could even reduce the risk of coronary disease.'

We also know that green tea helps blood circulation. A recent study published in the European Journal of Cardiovascular Prevention and Rehabilitation by Dr Nikolaos Alexopoulos and colleagues at the 1st Cardiology Department, Athens Medical School, found that green tea has a short-term beneficial effect on the large arteries, after using ultrasound scanning to measure the performance of the brachial artery.

100g Green tea nutrition information
Calories 6, Sugar 0%, Iron 0%, Vitamin C 0%

Yin and Yang score
Yang + Yin ++

Relation to Organs
Lungs, Heart, Spleen and Liver

WU-LONG TEA

You can drink 2-3 cups every day. Do not drink it after 6pm, as it might disrupt sleep due to its Yang energy boost.

Wu-long means 'black dragon' in Chinese – a reference to the tea leaves' unique resemblance to the curling body of mythical Chinese dragons. It refers to a method of production that produces a tea somewhere between oxidised black tea and non-oxidised green tea. This is why they are sometimes known as semi-oxidised and in China 'blue' teas.

The best wu-long tea is from Wuyi shan of China's Fujian province on the south-eastern coast. Tea innovations have been taking place here for more than 1000 years. The Wuyi shan acts as a protective barrier against the inflow of cold air from the northwest and retains warm moist air originating from the sea. As a result, the area has a humid climate with high rainfall and common fogs. Lower altitudes experience annual temperatures in the range from 12 °C to 18 °C. Cooler, wetter conditions prevail at higher altitudes and winters can be snowy on the highest peaks.

In Traditional Chinese medicine

Wu-long tea is a Yang energy source, with a reddish or brownish colour, and produces an amber to dark red tea water. The taste is sweet and fragrant, belonging to the spleen, liver and kidneys.

It increases Yang energy, and helps body function and

strengthens the body's organs and system, preventing fatigue and weakness.

- It especially helps the spleen to function to treat bloating and gas.
- It helps the liver function to act on fatty, oily food and alcohol problems, protecting damage to the body from toxins.
- It helps kidney function to quickly remove waste and unwanted water, ridding you of water retention.

So, it helps with weight loss and anti-ageing. It has been used for thousands of years. Long term drinking of wu-long tea will help the body detoxify, preventing constipation.

The health benefits are:

- Boosting Yang energy
- Helping weight loss
- Helping the body to detox
- Helping the immune system
- Helping with metabolism
- Helping with anti-ageing

Wu-long tea contains caffeine, which works by stimulating the central nervous system, heart, and muscles. Wu-long tea also contains theophylline and theobromine, which are chemicals similar to caffeine. This is why it is often said to sharpen thinking skills and improve mental alertness, while also thought to prevent cancer, tooth decay, osteoporosis and helping in obesity, diabetes and high cholesterol.

A study published by the US National Library of Medicine, National Institute of Health says 'Black tea contains mainly thearubigins, theaflavins, flavonols and catechins. The total polyphenol content of green and black teas is similar, but with different types of flavonoids present due to the degree of oxidation during processing'. The study also concluded that all catechins help metabolism and are cancer preventive.

100g Wu-long tea nutrition information
Calories 1, Sugar 0%, Iron 0%, Vitamin C 0%

Yin and Yang score
Yang ++ Yin ++

Relation to Organs
Spleen, Liver, Heart, Kidneys and Lungs

JASMINE TEA

You can drink 2-3 cups of jasmine tea each day. Do not drink it after 6pm, as it might disrupt sleep due to its Yang energy boost.

Jasmine tea is any tea (green, black or white etc.) that is then mixed with jasmine blossoms (a special scent, favoured by Chinese women). Its benefit depend on the original tea base, so the information below is related to the jasmine flower itself.

The jasmine flower only releases its fragrance at night after the sun has set and especially when the moon is waxing towards fullness. There are different colours of jasmine, such as slight yellowish white, blue, deep yellow, etc. as well as seasonal variations. Summer jasmine needs a fertile spot that is moist and well-drained, be it in a pot, garden or open space. Clay garden soil with a moderate level of fertility that is in full sun is the perfect condition for it to grow. The sunnier the spot, the better and more fragrant the scent.

Each individual jasmine plant should be kept at least eight feet apart in order to save the later growth of the plant from jamming together. Feeding leaf moulds to the soil makes it even better, as well as plenty of water during the summer months.

In Traditional Chinese medicine
The jasmine flower is a mainly Yin energy source, and its taste is rather mellow with a slight honey tinge.

- It helps the body detox, it helps the digestive system and it is relaxing.
- It treats liver disease (hepatitis) and liver pain due to cirrhosis.
- It treats abdominal pain due to severe diarrhoea (dysentery).
- It is also used to cause relaxation (as a sedative).

100g Jasmine flower nutrition information
Calories 56.2, Sugar 0%, Iron 4%, Vitamin C 1%

Yin and Yang score

Yin + Yang ++

Relations to Organs

Liver, Spleen and Kidneys

CAMOMILE TEA

This is spelt in two ways: chamomile (American English) or camomile (British English).
You can drink 3-5 cups per day.

Camomile plants can be bought ready-grown for planting in spring, though Roman camomile can be planted from seeds. Sow seeds in late spring then place in a warm spot. When the seedlings are large enough they can be planted in the garden in a sunny position, or kept in the pot. Camomile can be clipped regularly during the growing season; gather newly-opened flowers in summer and early autumn for tea making.

In Traditional Chinese medicine

Camomile tea is a Yin energy source mainly and Yang (Qi) energy source.

- It eliminates excessive heat from the lungs, liver and heart.
- It helps the liver, calming, relaxing and detoxing. Drinking camomile is especially beneficial when you are stressed, anxious or depressed. It also helps the heart, reducing stress-related heart rate problems.

- It helps spleen function to digest easily.
- It also helps the lungs to function and can treat skin disorder or eyes infection, i.e. you'll see great results if you use camomile tea to wash your eyes or skin disorder area once or twice a day.

The camomile flower is often used in the treatment of chest colds, sore throats, gum inflammation (gingivitis), insomnia, stomach ulcers and skin problems – camomile tea has the same function.

Its primary health benefits are:

- Detoxifying
- Improving the immune system
- Helping the body relax
- Anti-ageing

The US National Library of Medicine National Institute Health published an article saying, 'The dried flowers of chamomile contain many terpenoids and flavonoids contributing to its medicinal properties. Chamomile preparations are commonly used for many human ailments such as hay fever, inflammation, muscle spasms, menstrual disorders, insomnia, ulcers, wounds, gastrointestinal disorders, rheumatic pain, and hemorrhoids. Essential oils of chamomile are used extensively in cosmetics and aromatherapy'. For more information visit www.ncbi.nlm.nih.gov.com

Studies by the American Chemical Society's Journal of Agricultural and Food Chemistry found that 'drinking the tea was associated with a significant increase in urinary levels of hippurate, known as phenolics, some of which have been associated with increased antibacterial activity. Drinking the tea also was associated with an increase in urinary levels of glycine, an amino acid that has been shown to relieve muscle spasms'.

The University of Maryland Medical Centre also discovered that 'German chamomile reduces inflammation, speeds wound healing, reduces muscle spasms, and serves as a mild sedative to help with sleep. Test tube studies have shown that chamomile can kill bacteria, fungus, and viruses.'

100g Camomile tea nutrition information
Calories 1, Sugar 0%, Iron 0%, Vitamin C 0%

Yin and Yang score
Yang + Yin ++

Relation to Organs
Lungs, Liver, Kidneys, Spleen and Heart

LEMON TEA
You can drink 3-5 cups of lemon tea every day.
Lemon tree species (Citrus limon) is a species of small evergreen tree in the flowering plant family Rutaceae, native to Asia. It grows in tropical and subtropical humid regions; it flourishes well in temperate and tropical environments, whereas, cold and frosty conditions can

affect their growth adversely. Stems and branches often have sharp, stout thorns but the fully-grown plant bears fragrant, white flowers with a short stem. It tolerates drought, is highly sensitive to frost and unhappy in shade for more than six months.

The distinctive sour taste of lemon juice makes it a key ingredient in making tea, cocktails or as an accompaniment to seafood, and even salad. Lemon has been wildly used in diet food and drinks, natural cleaning products, health products, and also in weight loss, detoxing, and anti-ageing programmes as well.

In Traditional Chinese medicine

Lemon tea is both a Yang energy source and Yin energy source. It is a little bitter and sour, and affects the body's energy of Qi and Yin. It is the No.1 fruit and can have strong medical usage. It is a good source for maintaining function in all organs.

- It helps the liver to regulate liver Qi, helping treat the causes of anxiety, depression and headaches.
- It helps the spleen's Qi, clearing toxins and speeding up the passage of fatty or oily food to help with digestion.
- It helps the lung Qi, increasing lung strength, bringing oxygen to all the body systems.
- It helps heart Qi, regulating blood circulation.
- It helps in kidney Qi, combatting water retention

It also helps Yin energy, calming and relaxing, reducing

excessive heat toxin. It reduces excessive heat that causes skin problems, relieving aches in muscles and joints, sore throats and flu, etc.

Its primary health benefits are:

- Cleansing body toxin
- Helping the digestive system
- Assisting in weight loss
- Improving the immune system
- Preventing kidney stones

The lemon has the lowest amount of calories in the citrus fruits group but the highest level of vitamin C (ascorbic acid). Ascorbic acid is both water-soluble and a natural anti-oxidant. It prevents scurvy and helps the body fight against infectious agents and seek out harmful, pro-inflammatory free radicals from the blood. Citric acid is also a natural preservative, aids in smooth digestion, and helps dissolve kidney stones. Furthermore, it contains a variety of phytochemicals that work as immune modulators, free-radical scavengers and are anti-inflammatory.

A recent study by the BBC found that 'some evidence has linked vitamin C (or ascorbic acid) and flavonoid to improvements in skin. Vitamin C is known to help the body produce collagen, which contributes to the strength of the skin'.

100g Lemon nutrition information
Calories 29, Sugar 4.2g, Iron 4%, Vitamin C 88%, Calcium 3%

LILY LI HUA

Yin and Yang score
Yang +++ Yin +++++

Relation to Organs
Liver, Heart, Kidneys, Spleen and Lungs

MINT TEA

You can drink 2-3 cups of mint tea each day.
Mint (Menthe) is known for its highly aromatic leaves, used in cooking or to make tea. Mint can also be used to control insect pests in the garden. While it does not kill them, its powerful scent can keep pests away from desirable plants and host beneficial insect predators to help control the pest population.

Mint is a very interesting plant. It has a high medical value, and can be found in many healthy products, such as toothpastes, chewing gums and breath fresheners. It is also used in medicine treatment for cold or flu and sore throat.

In Traditional Chinese medicine
Mint tea is mainly a Yin energy source – it has a cool character, and is bitter and spicy. It mainly contains Yin energy, reducing excessive heat toxins and tension.

- It helps the liver, releasing stress caused by anxiety, depression, sleeplessness, and tension headaches.
- It helps to relax the heart and clear heat from the liver.

99

- It help in skin disorders, or chronic eye infections and inflammation.
- It also helps with detoxification, especially important when you eat too much oily or fatty food.

Its primary health benefits are:

- Helping the body relax
- Helping the immune system
- Assisting in body weight loss
- Detoxification

Mint is rich in iron. In the human body hemoglobin represents about two-thirds of the body's iron. If you don't have enough iron, your body can't make enough healthy oxygen-carrying red blood cells. A lack of red blood cells is called iron deficiency anemia. Without healthy red blood cells, your body can't get enough oxygen. This is one reason when you drink mint tea often, you will have increased energy.

Mint also contains high levels of calcium. Calcium is essential for the health of your bones and teeth, but it also affects your muscles, hormones, nerve function, and ability to form blood clots. Plus, research has suggested – although not yet confirmed – that calcium may help other problems like PMS, high blood pressure, and possibly fight weight gain.

Mint is also rich in vitamins C and A. It is a powerful antioxidant, helping the body form and maintain connective tissue, including bones, blood vessels, and skin.

100g Mint nutrition information

Calories 70, Sugar 0%, Iron 28%, Vitamin C 53%, Vitamin A 85%, Calcium 24%

Yin and Yang score

Yang +   Yin ++++

Relation to Organs

Liver, Heart, Bones and Skin

GINGER TEA

You can drink 2-3 cups of ginger tea 2-3 cups per day.
Ginger tea uses the root from ginger plants. Ginger can planted in a pot, garden or field. In warm climates, it prefers shade for most of the day. In cooler climates, you can grow ginger in containers placed in the sun. When ginger is grown in pots, add fresh soil as more stems emerge and the plants grow taller. Nutrients from the fresh soil help feed the plants, but container-grown plants also need regular feeding with a balanced organic fertilizer through the first half of summer, while they are growing rapidly and producing new leaves.

In Traditional Chinese medicine

Ginger tea is a Yang energy source, with a warm and spicy taste.

- It boosts the spleen's Yang energy, helping to treat gas and bloating.

- It boosts the stomach's Yang energy, helping with loss of appetite or stomach pain and vomiting problems,
- It boosts the kidneys' Yang energy, treating poor blood circulation, tiredness and water retention.

Ginger tea can help regulate Qi free movement and treat Qi or blood blockage, such as stomach pain, period pain, headache and hair loss. Traditionally people used fresh ginger slices directly to areas of hair loss, stimulating the hair gland to increase blood circulation. Ginger tea also helps chronic irritable bowel movement syndrome (IBS).

Lots of health products in China and the West contain ginger, such as ginger tonic water, ginger juice, ginger detox tea, ginger beer and anti-dandruff shampoo, including the popular Zhang guang 101 (章光101) shampoo in China for hair loss.

Its primary health benefits are:

- Helping the digestive system
- Helping to boost energy
- Detoxification
- Helping hair growth
- Helping the immune system

Studies have often found that ginger helps the metabolism, antioxidant activity, is anti- cancer, and is anti-inflammatory. Taking a small amount of ginger daily is also said to significantly reduce several liver enzymes, inflammatory cytokines, and insulin resistance.

Another important fact is that ginger contains 10% DV of magnesium – double compared to other vegetables. Magnesium helps maintain normal muscle and nerve function, keeps the heart rhythm steady, supports a healthy immune system, and keeps bones strong. Magnesium also helps regulate blood sugar levels, promoting normal blood pressure.

100g Ginger nutrition information

Calories 80, Sugar 1.7g, Iron 3%, Vitamin C 8%, Vitamin B6 10%, Magnesium 10%

Yin and Yang score

Yang +++   Yin +

Relation to Organs

Heart, Liver, Spleen, Digestive System, Bones and Hair

Other teas that can help with weight loss are as follows:
- White Tea
- Pu erg Tea
- Raspberry Tea
- Chickweed Tea
- Feign Tea
- Detoxing Tea

FRUITS

In China, fruits are fundamental to the Yin and Yang balance and philosophy. In the West, fruits provide calories and minerals. However, in past times, people ate fruit that was only available locally, rather than what was good for them. Nowadays, because we have access to foods from across the world, we have so much more choice. But different fruits have different levels of nutrition, and it's good to know what fruits are suitable for your personal health needs.

The nutritional value of fruit depends on many factors – the climate where they are grown, such as heat, dryness, soil, temperature, time for maturation and levels of pollution at the source. As a rule, fruits grown high in the mountains are better than those grown in lower levels; fruits that take longer to grow have more nutritional value than fast-growing fruits. High mountain fruits are always better than others.

So how do Chinese people distinguish fruits as Yin or Yang? In general, fruits are the same as vegetables or other natural food sources but we follow the rules below:

- **Colour**: deep colour is Yang, light colour is Yin; red colour is Yang, green colour is Yin.
- **Taste**: sweet taste is Yang, bitter taste is Yin; spicy is Yang and sour is Yin.
- **Texture and size**: hard texture is Yang, soft texture is Yin; large size is Yang, small size is Yin.

Each fruit can have a Yin and a Yang benefit, especially if a fruit has more than one attribute and taste. In this case it will have more nutritional benefits, i.e. strawberries can help in increasing Yin energy and your blood flow but also help Yang energy, and all your bodily functions.

Similarly, watermelon is Yin energy due to the high amount of water it contains, but it is also sweet and red in colour, so it also has Yang energy.

Hopefully, after reading the book, your knowledge of Yin and Yang food principles will increase, helping you to make better choices. For example, I've often heard people say that watermelon has a high sugar content so it is not good for weight loss. But honestly, watermelon has less sugar and calories than an apple does, and a higher level of vitamin C as well. It also contains 92% water which is essential in everyday life, as long as you balance the amount you have.

How much fruit is good for you? That really depends on your diet and preferences. But always make sure to balance your vegetables, fruit and water intake every day.

APPLE

You can eat 2-3 medium size apples per day.
Apples have a great reputation in terms of health benefits, with the old saying being 'an apple a day, keeps the doctor away'. They are easily grown, cheap and full of nutritious benefits.

Apple trees grow pretty much all year round, easily surviving a harsh winter. As the seasons change to spring, the apple tree blossoms and bears fruit, and the tree's temperature tolerance rises. An apple tree's temperature tolerance depends upon what stage of bloom the tree is in. The best apples grow in well-drained soils. Apples succeed best in regions where the trees experience uninterrupted rest in winter and plenty of sun for good colour. They can be grown above the sea level and cope with heavy rainfall.

In Traditional Chinese medicine

Apples are mainly a Yang energy source but they also have Yin energy, as they are both sweet and slightly sour and warm. It helps all of the bodily functions and organs in Qi and Yin.

- It helps the spleen's Qi, increasing its digestive function and helping with bloating or gas.
- It helps the liver Qi function in detoxification, especially with foods that are fatty, oily or there is alcohol-toxic damage in the body.
- It helps the lung's Qi energy, improving the body's oxygen level and removing toxic gas.
- It helps the Yang energy of the heart and the kidneys, helping to keep the heart healthy and to detox the kidneys.
- It is Yin toxin and nourishment, good for skin tone and your joint flexibility.

Its primary health benefits are:

- Helping the digestive system
- Helping the liver with detoxification
- Helping in weight loss
- Improving the body's immunity
- Preventing constipation

Apples contain a certain type of fibre called pectin which is found between the cell walls of plants and is classified as soluble fibre. Soluble fibre has been shown to slow down digestion by attracting water and forming a gel which ultimately helps you feel fuller longer. Additionally, it provide vitamins such as C, A and folate, as well as minerals, including potassium and phosphorous. Vitamin A is a powerful antioxidant to help resist infection and scavenge free radicals that cause inflammation, and free radical damage cause by pollution, cigarette smoke and UV rays.

Lots of published articles have found that apples help the liver detox, just like using a mop to clean up mess on the kitchen floor. The main reason for this is that apples keep the liver rich in pectin, the soluble fibre that helps remove toxins and cholesterol from the blood. Apples are also rich in malic acid, a naturally cleansing nutrient that removes carcinogens and other toxins from the blood. Granny Smith apples are especially rich in malic acid. Health experts recommended eliminating or reducing animal foods to care for your liver, just as much as they advise reducing alcohol consumption, refined sugar, excess caffeine, and processed foods.' (Source: www.onegreenplants.org)

100g Apple nutrition information
Calories 52, Sugar 10g, Iron 0%, Vitamin C 7%, Vitamin B 6 0%

Yin and Yang score

Yang ++ Yin ++++

Relation to Organs

Lungs, Liver, Heart, Kidneys and Spleen

WATERMELON

You can eat 4-6 medium-sized pieces of watermelon per day.

Watermelon plants grow from the middle of spring through to summer. They need a long and warm growing season of at least 70 to 85 days, depending on the variety, to produce sweet fruit. They grow best when daytime temperatures fall between 70 and 80 degrees Fahrenheit, and night-time temperatures fall between 65 and 70 degrees Fahrenheit.

In Traditional Chinese medicine

Watermelon is a mainly Yin energy source, but it is a little Qi (part of Yang) energy source as well. It contains 92% water, and is sweet and cool. It is excellent to refresh the body system and in reducing excessive heat. It helps all organs, and treats sore throats and dehydration.

- It helps the heart's Yin energy and helps to reduce a fast heart rate due to toxins or excessive heat. It nourishes your skin and other body tissues, helping the body to rehydrate, flushing your system and removing excessive heat.

- It helps the spleen's Qi energy and eases digestion, removing toxic produced normally by your body's system.
- It helps the kidney function in detoxing and works almost like an air-conditioner to pump out body heat and hot air, replacing it with new air and fresh cold water. It really is one of the best fruits to eat in the hot weather. Lots of health products are made from watermelon, including special powders for toothache and mouth ulcers.

It is one of the most popular fruits in the diet world and medical health field.

Its main health benefits are

- Helping with detoxification
- Preventing constipation
- Helping heart health
- Helping anti-ageing
- Helping in weight loss
- Helping stress relief

Watermelon is rich in amino acid, which helps to relax blood vessels and improve circulation. It is widely found to reduce blood pressure, a major risk factor in heart disease, so it really could be a lifesaver. In fact, a recent study by Florida State University found that post-menopausal women experienced improved cardiovascular health after eating a diet rich in watermelon.

100g Watermelon nutrition information
Calories 30, Sugar 6g, Iron 1%, Vitamin C 13%

Yin and Yang score
Yang ++ Yin +++++

Relation to Organs
Lungs, Spleen, Liver, Heart and Kidneys

KIWI

You can eat 2-4 medium size kiwis per day.
Kiwi fruit used to be very rare in China because it was so expensive – it was only eaten by the royal family or the very wealthy. The main reason for this is because it grows in such special climates, in mountainous regions 800 to 2900 metres high. It is native to north-central and eastern China, and the first recorded description of it dates back to the 12th century China during the Song dynasty. Cultivation of the kiwi fruit spread from China in the early 20th century to New Zealand, then gradually started being farmed in Italy and America (in America it is called the Chinese gooseberry). It really does have such wonderful nutritional benefits, and has been valued for its medicinal properties since ancient times.

In Traditional Chinese medicine
Kiwi is a good source of both Yin and Yang energy. It is sweet with a dark brown fur coating, and the inner fruit looks like green crystal, with a white centre and black seeds.

- It helps Yang energy and has benefits for all body functions. It helps the liver the liver to function and regulate Qi and Yang; it helps the nervous system, helping you to focus; it helps the heart's Qi and Yang level, increasing strength and preventing clotting; it helps the spleen's Qi and Yang, increasing digestive functions; it helps the kidneys' and the lungs' Qi and Yang.
- It contains Yin energy, beneficial for the regeneration of the skin, bones and ligament; it helps fertility function; and it is also thought to good for the memory.
- It is one of the finest fruits due to its function in detoxing and combatting skin damage by sun or pollution.

Its primary health benefits are below:

- Helping body detoxification
- Boost energy
- Boost immune system
- Helping in anti-ageing
- Helping slimming

Kiwi is the king of vitamin C – I really couldn't believe my eyes when I first realised – and contains nearly 22 times more than an apple, nearly 12 times than watermelon, 14 times than peach, 1.5 times than strawberries, 2 times than an orange, and 3 times than a whole pineapple.

There is iron higher level as well, in the same amount

of fruit. It has the same iron as an apple and orange, 2 times the level of watermelon and peaches, only strawberries have the same. Additionally, it has a high iron content and also contains vitamin K, vitamin E, folate, and potassium, as well as being a good source of fibre.

It can be credited with multiple benefits due to the fact it neutralises free radicals and can help prevent cell damage and inflammation, potentially preventing things like cancer and is a heart-healthy superstar. A suggested one kiwi a day can provide a lower risk of stroke, blood clots and cardiovascular diseases. The potassium in kiwi fruit can also help to lower blood pressure, counteract sodium in the body and is a vasodilator, relaxing the blood vessels throughout the body.

100g Kiwi nutrition information
Calories 61, Sugar 9%, Iron 2%, Vitamin C 54%, Vitamin B-6 5%

Yin and Yang score
Yang ++++ Yin +++++

Relation to Organs
Lungs, Liver, Heart, Kidneys and Spleen

ASIAN PEARS

You can eat 2-3 medium size Chinese pears per day.
Pears have several types, but I'm going to refer to the Asian pears due to their historical medical effect. The

Asian pears' scientific name is *pyrus species* and there are three types of Asian pears – round or roundish-flat fruit with green to yellow skin, round or roundish-flat fruit with yellow to brown skin and bronze to gold russet (little dots), or pear-shaped with green skin or brown skin and bronze russet.

Asian Pears have beautiful flowers in spring, and traditionally require cross-pollination, with a female and male tree planted next to each other – doing this provides better tasting fruit and they will bear more fruits in each tree. They re harvested in late summer to autumn, but can vary based on variety and location. Asian pears like full sun, tolerate very little shade, and need medium soil moisture.

In Traditional Chinese medicine

Asian pears are a source of both Qi, Yin and Yang energy. They are excellent for the lungs and the detoxing system.

- It helps the lung's Qi, helping to remove toxins and toxic water when we breathe out.
- It helps the lungs' Yin, releasing dryness caused by coughs, sore throat, or irritated skin.
- It helps the heart's Qi and Yin.
- It helps the spleen's ability to digest food.

Chinese people will steam a pear with one tbsp. of yellow crystal sugar to help with chronic coughs and asthma.
Its primary health benefits are:

- Improving immune system
- Helping skin problems
- Helping in weight loss
- Helping constipation
- Helping detoxing

Asian pears are low in calories and vitamin C, as in traditional Chinese green tea or wu-long tea as well. Due to its low calorie and sugar level, it is great to eat when trying to lose weight, avoid hunger and help in diabetes.

A recent study found that pears may regulate alcohol metabolism and also protect against ulcers. They are also high in fibre, low in calories and contain a number of micronutrients that are important for blood, bone and cardiovascular health.

100g Asian pears nutrition information

Calories 42, Sugar 7g, Iron 0%, Vitamin C 6%, Magnesium 2%, Vitamin B-6 0%

Yin and Yang score

Yang + Yin +++

Relation to Organs

Lungs, Spleen, Liver and Kidneys

STRAWBERRIES

You can eat 10-20 medium-sized strawberries per day. Strawberries are best planted in the spring or late summer, avoiding the cold weather of late autumn and winter. They can grow in pots, gardens or open space and will fruit 60 days after planting. They prefer a sunny and sheltered position in fertile, free-draining soil. However, summer-fruiting and perpetual-fruiting strawberries may not grow so well in the shade.

In Traditional Chinese medicine

Strawberries are both a Yin and Qi (part of Yang) energy source. It is Qi (Yang) energy due to its red colour and sweetness, but it is Yin energy as it is juicy and contains a high level of water.

- It helps the body's Yang energy, e.g. the liver Qi that regulates the liver and the spleen's Qi digestive function to produce less toxins. It also helps the kidneys' Qi and Jing (special vital energy) that reduces water retention.
- It helps the body's Yin energy, e.g. increasing nourishment to the skin and helping the skin hydrate, preventing skin damage from the sun and pollution. It's also a good fruit to help fertility function.

Its primary health benefits are:

- Helping in weight loss

- Anti-inflammation
- Helping in detoxing
- Helping prevent heart problems
- Anti-ageing

Strawberries really are one of the finest fruits I have studied, and are considered a 'diamond' in healthy food and weight loss. It is low in calories and sugar, high in vitamin C, with a rich and soft texture. It really is perfect to help in weight loss.

100g Strawberries nutrition information
Calories 32, Sugar 4.66g, Iron 2%, Vitamin C 98%, Vitamin B-6 0%

Yin and Yang score
Yang +++ Yin +++++

Relation to Organs
Lungs, Liver, Heart, Kidneys and Spleen

PINEAPPLES
You can eat 2-3 medium-sized pieces per day.
Pineapples grow in very special conditions and with very little water. They also need well-aerated soils. Good drainage is essential because poor drainage leads to a weak root system, which makes the plant more susceptible to diseases. Temperature is the most important climatic factor affecting productivity. Because of the warm

climates it grows in, it is packed full of beneficial dietary fibre and bromelain (an enzyme).

In Traditional Chinese medicine

Qi (Pineapple is a good Yin and Yang) energy source compared with other fruits, as they have fibrous flesh that is yellow in colour, and a vibrant tropical flavour that balances the tastes of sweet and tart. Its texture is both hard and soft.

It is particularly beneficial for the spleen, lungs and kidneys, increasing their Qi and Yin. It helps in breathing strength, reducing dry coughs, as well as preventing skin damage from sun and water retention.

Its primary health benefits are:

- Helping in weight loss
- Preventing constipation
- Helping body detoxing
- Helping in anti-ageing

Pineapple has a high enzyme content, specifically bromelain, helping to break down toxins in the body to prepare them for elimination and as a result, you feel better and digestion even improves. It is high in vitamin C, so excellent for your liver and can improve your overall immune function. Best of all, pineapple is also high in potassium which helps flush wastes from the body and supports overall water balance.

Pineapple reduces swelling, and pineapple juice has been known to help reduce coughing. Additionally, it contains the bromelin enzyme which helps the lungs remove debris and detox naturally.

100g Pineapple nutrition information

Calories 50, Sugar 10g, Iron 1%, Vitamin C 79%, Vitamin B-6 5%

Yin and Yang score

Yang +++ Yin ++++

Relation to Organs

Lungs, Liver, Digestive System and Spleen

ORANGES

You can eat 2-3 medium-sized oranges per day.

Oranges are one of the finest fruits you can eat, providing energy, cleansing and helping with all bodily functions.

The orange family consists of sweet oranges (Citrus sinensis) and sour oranges (Citrus aurantium), growing in tropical and subtropical climates with hot summers and mild winters this juicy fruit is produced. It is a most beautiful tree and good for the environment.

In Traditional Chinese medicine

Orange is a strong Yang energy source and Yin energy source, with a sweet-sour citric taste, a little bit juicy with bumpy texture. It really does balance all the organs in Yang, Qi, Yin and blood.

- Especially in strengthening the whole body's Yang and Qi energy, improving all organ function.
- It helps the Yin and blood level, helping the body to detox and preventing body stiffness, clotting and memory loss.
- It is an excellent fruit to prevent body damage due to its detoxing ability. It is excellent in helping the skin heal from sun or pollution damage.

Its primary health benefits are:

- Helping the body to detox
- Helping the body boost energy
- Helping heart strength
- Boosting the immune system
- Helping with weight loss
- Helping in anti-ageing

Oranges are favoured in both Chinese and Western culture due to their low calories and high levels of vitamin C – 1 medium size (131 grams) orange contains 13% fibre, 10% folate, 9%, vitamin B1 and 5% calcium, all essential to health and nutrition needs. Oranges are well known as having 12 times the amount of vitamin C than apples, which is a powerful antioxidant, protecting the immune system and disarming free radicals that cause cell damage. Their abundance of folate reduces levels of homocysteine, the cardiovascular risk factor, which can build up in our blood, while their store of potassium helps lower blood pressure.

A recent study even found that oranges strengthen our emotional wellbeing, and a compound found in citrus fruits is thought to lower the risk of stroke in women.

100g Orange nutrition information

Calories 47, Sugar 9g, Iron 0%, Vitamin C 88%, Vitamin B-6 5%

Yin and Yang score

Yang +++ Yin +++++

Relation to Organs

Lungs, Liver, Heart, Kidneys and Spleen

Other fruits that can help weight loss:

- Avocado
- Blackberries
- Blueberries
- Cranberries
- Lemons
- Limes
- Nectarines
- Peaches
- Pumpkin
- Tomatoes

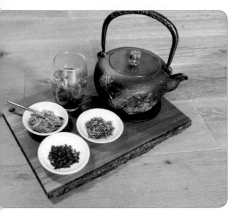

Green tea, wu-long tea and long jing tea – key to your A.B.C.D rotation.

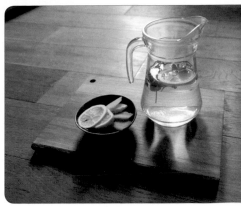

Cold water to accompany each meal.

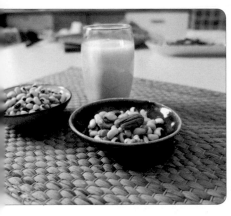

Blended milk and nuts are a perfect way to start the day.

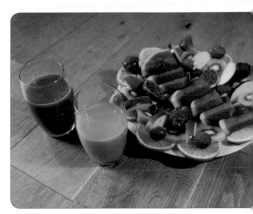

Mixed fruit juice is perfect for breakfast.

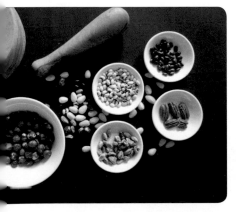

Dried nuts, like pistachios and almonds are great to keep you satisfied throughout the day.

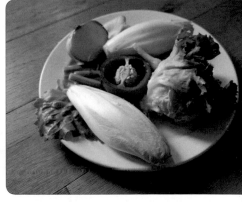

A key selection of vegetables, to be eaten at every meal.

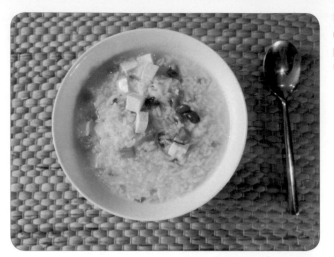

Rice porridge with mixed beans – see page 157 for the recipe.

Chinese rice porridge – see page 153 for the recipes.

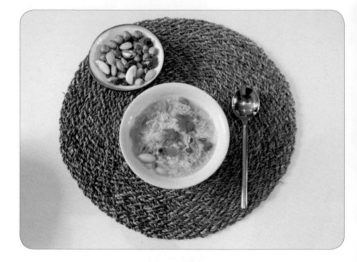

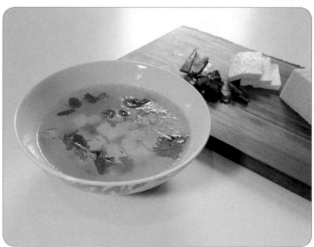

Soups and porridges are perfect for breakfast, lunch and dinner, and are so quick to make.

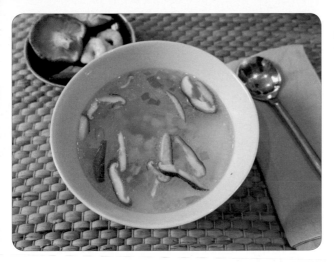

Prawn and mushroom soup – see page 225 for the recipe.

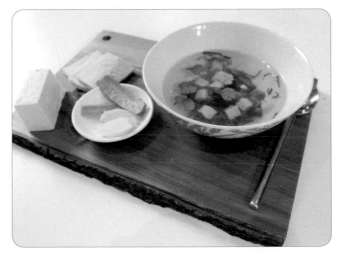

Tofu and dry seaweed soup – see page 177 for the recipe.

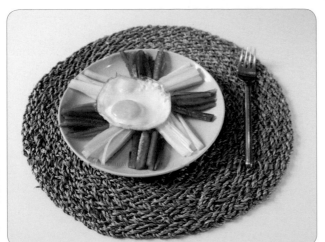

Look for my easy egg recipes on page 162.

Black fungus is a great source of both Yin and Yang energy.

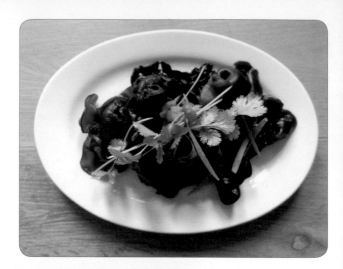

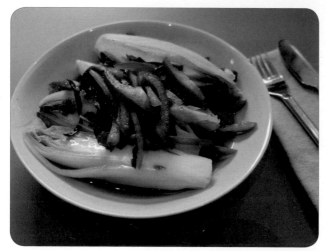

Great Grub Club – see page 186 for the recipe.

Asparagus and carrot is a perfect lunchtime meal – see page 190 for the recipe.

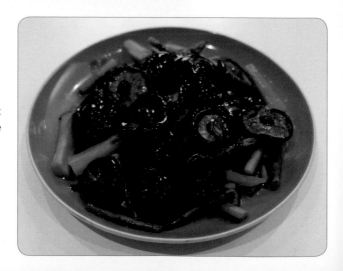

Four Season – see page 232 for the recipe.

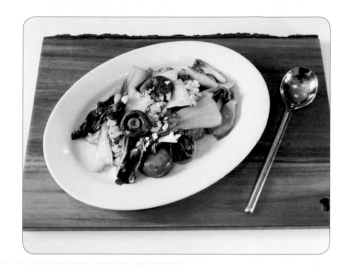

Tofu and Shiitake Mushrooms – see page 192 for the recipe.

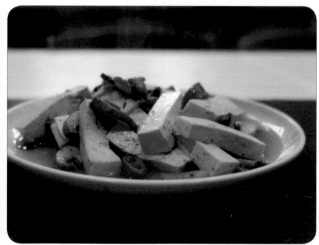

Aubergines make a delicious meal for vegans and vegetarians.

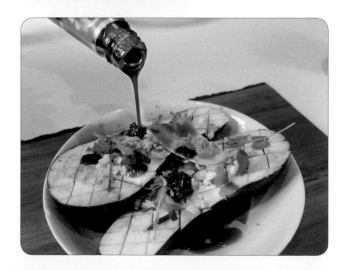

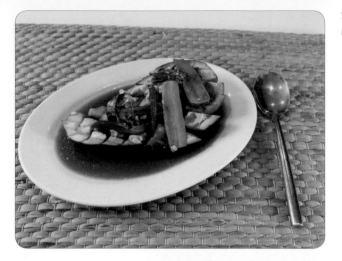

See page 141 for the recipes.

See page 141 for the recipes.

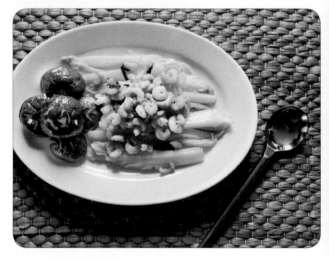

So many dishes can be made quickly and easily in the microwave, like Disney Beauty – see page 198 for the recipe.

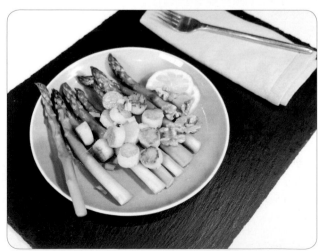

Season Greeting – see page 230 for the recipe.

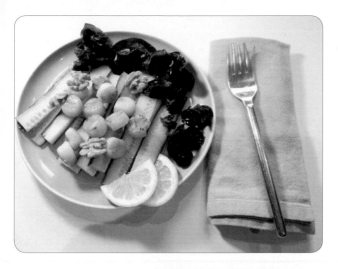

Many of the recipes can easily be adapted to add seafood and meat.

King of Speech – see page 201 for the recipe.

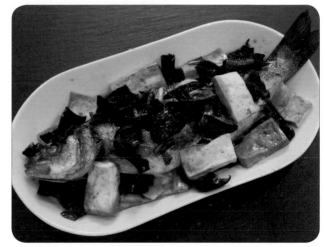

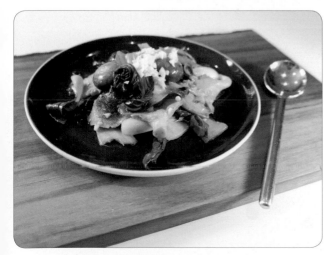

Pak choi with mushrooms and garlic is a perfect choice for any of the lunch and evening meals.

Middle Autumn –
see page 209 for
the recipe.

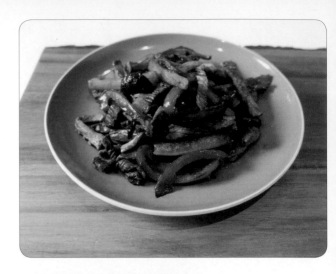

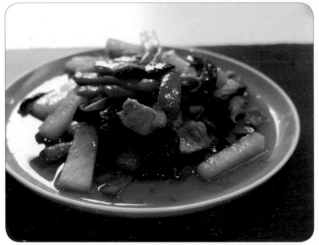

Chicken is a great
accompaniment
to so many of the
vegetable dishes.

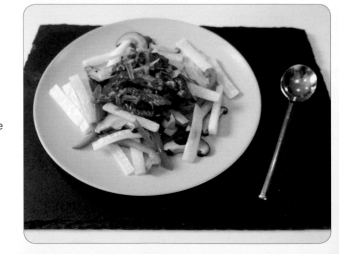

Amazing Concert –
see page 211 for the
recipe.

Vegetables

Generally speaking, the Chinese diet hasn't changed much in 3,000 years – we still eat to maintain the balance of Yin and Yang, and our body's natural balance.

In ancient times, people would eat vegetables that were grown locally, easily bought at the small markets in the villages or towns. This limited variety meant that there were less health problems, because we knew what kinds of food our body needed and that food was locally sourced. Nowadays, we can get all variety of vegetables from across the world at any time. Eating vegetables without knowledge of their nutritional value may cause you health problems. Here are steps to help you distinguish the Yin and Yang nutrition value of various vegetables in several ways:

- Colour: light is Yin, deep is Yang; green is Yin, red is Yang.
- Taste: Sweet and spicy vegetables are a Yang energy source; bitter, sour and salty are a Yin energy source.
- Texture: if a vegetable is hard or difficult to cook, it is Yang; otherwise it is Yin.
- Climate: if a vegetable is grown in full sun or hot weather, taking a long time to grow, it is Yang; otherwise it is Yin.

The seven vegetables I talk about in more detail all have something in common for the recipes, later in this book:

- They can be used in all types of recipes.
- They can be eaten on their own or as an accompaniment to a main dish.
- They are all good for weight loss, or your general wellbeing.
- They all contain their own sodium and sugar, which means that you can use less or no salt and sugar.

Tofu, black mushroom and black fungus play a double role as they have a 'meat' quality, which boosts Yang energy but they also enhance Yin energy, helping the body to repair and build muscle and bones etc.

WHITE RADISH

The radishes' scientific name is *Raphanus Sativus*. Its root belongs to the family of Brassica. There are 5 different type of radish: Red globe radishes (*Raphanus sativus*), white daikon, Spanish radishes, green radish and watermelon radishes. The most commonly used radishes are the red globe radishes and white daikon.

In the Chinese culture, the white radish is one of the healthiest vegetables. There is an old saying in Chinese culture: 'Radish and tofu is key to a guaranteed wellbeing and comfort, eating pungent radish and drinking hot tea, let the starved doctors beg on their knees.'

In Traditional Chinese medicine
Radishes are a Yin and Yang energy source. They are sweet and crispy with a crystal and watery texture, which

is helpful for the whole body. It is mainly beneficial in helping to increase body Qi and Yin.

- It helps body Qi, improving body function. The increase in spleen Qi also helps with releasing gas, relieving discomfort. It can also be used to treat stomach tension and pain due to food dyspeptic retention, help smooth Qi movement, and release Qi blockages that can cause abdominal pain.
- It improves the body's Yin energy, nourishment of skin, muscle, etc. It helps the body release water retention and removes toxic water from the lungs, spleen and kidneys. These are some of the reasons why it is so beneficial in aiding weight loss.
- It helps the liver and spleen function, digesting fatty food and alcohol. It helps to remove toxins fast and minimise toxic damage as well. Fatty foods and radishes are often eaten together, as it is comfortable on the stomach.

From the beginning of Traditional Chinese Medicine over 3,000 years ago till the present day, radishes have been medically used to remove gas after surgery and bring natural colon movement back. People who suffer from chronic stomach ulcers, gastritis, IBS (irritable bowel syndrome), are advised to eat radishes as it can help to improve some of the symptoms associated with the conditions.

Radishes help the body break down oily or fatty food, as well as animal fat. This is why Chinese people can often be seen cooking meat mixed with radishes.

It has the following health benefits:

- Helps the digestive system
- Helps to prevent weight gain
- Helps to reduce stress
- Helps the body to detox
- Helps to rid hunger and fat stored in the body

Radish is an excellent source of vitamin K, vitamin C and vitamin B6, all essential nutrition to maintaining and repairing the body's needs. It contains high levels of fibre and water, making it easy for the digestive system, metabolic function, and reducing gas produced.

100 gram White radish nutrition information
Calories 18, Sugar 2.5g, Iron 2%, Vitamin C 36%

Yin and Yang score
Yin +++++ Yang +++

Relation to Organs
Lungs, Spleen, Liver, Digestive System and Heart

CUCUMBER

The cucumber's scientific name is Cucumis sativus and it belongs to the same botanical family. It is a popular vegetable used for weight loss and is used by many companies in both weight loss products as well as a beauty agent.

In Traditional Chinese medicine

Cucumber is one of the finest Qi (part of Yang energy) and Yin energy source; cool and sweet with a neutral taste, it is soft and watery making it easy for the body to process. It is good for the lungs, liver, kidneys, spleen, and nourishment of body Qi and Yin.

- It helps the body's Qi to improve function; ie. it helps the lungs function and clear body toxin. Qi helps the spleen to digest food regularly and remove waste quickly; and it helps the kidneys to reduce water retention.
- It helps the body's Yin, i.e. helps detoxify any toxins, such as skin disorders or damaged and irritated skin; it plays a part in keeping the skin smooth, joints flexible and muscles firm.
- It replenishes the skin and removes toxins and damage caused by the sun or pollution.
- The body of a cucumber has a watery texture and the seeds are easy to digest. As it is a watery body it flushes toxic water from the body's system and reduces water retention, all functions that help weight gain.

Its primary benefits are the following:

- Helping detoxification
- Helping in weight loss
- Helping in anti-ageing
- Helping the immune system

Studies have shown that the cucumber is very high in water content and very low in calories. The cucumber has a cleansing action within the body by removing accumulated pockets of old waste materials and chemical toxins. Fresh cucumber juice is used for nourishing the skin, hence why it is popularly used in beauty products; it gives a soothing effect against skin irritations and reduces swelling. Cucumber also has the power to relax and alleviate pain from sunburns. The seeds also have a cooling effect on the body and they can be used to prevent constipation.

100 gram Cucumber nutrition information
Calories 16, Sugar 1.7g, Iron 1%, Vitamin C 4%

Yin and Yang score
Yin +++++ Yang ++

Relation to Organs
Liver, Spleen, Digestive System, Lungs and Kidneys

CELERY

Celery, which is scientifically known as *Apium graveolens*, is another important vegetable for weight loss. It has a special flavour to keep unhealthy germs away from the body.

Celery is an easy to plant vegetable which is fast growing. It likes fertile soil, cool temperatures, and constant moisture. Celery is a heavy feeder and requires lots of water, during the entire growing season, especially during hot, dry weather.

In Traditional Chinese medicine

Celery has high levels of Yang and Yin energy. It is aromatic, sweetish, crunchy, acidic and neutral. It is vital for the liver, heart, kidneys, stomach, spleen and has incredible benefits for Qi, Yang and Yin.

- It provides the body system in Yang energy. It benefits all organs, the immune system, muscles and bone. It helps the body in Yin energy, in rejuvenation, repairing and general body function.
- It boost the spleen's Qi energy and helps the digestive system function on a regular basis, and it also helps to prevent constipation. It helps the kidneys' Qi energy to prevent water retention.
- It boosts the body's Yin energy and protects our body system environment. Its speciality is reducing toxin heat from our own system or food produced. It can cure skin conditions such as infections and inflammation as well as keep germs away from our gut or urine track. The leaf can be boiled with water and used to wash damaged skin. It can calm and reduce tension in the body which offers an explanation for why it is believed to reduce high blood pressure
- It can speed up the time that fatty food is digested

and got rid of, reducing the amount of toxin in our body.

Its primary health benefits are as below:

- Helping in weight loss
- Helping reduce high cholesterol
- Protecting the body's natural environment
- Helping the immune system

Celery contains antioxidants, vitamin k, potassium, folate and vitamin B6 and dietary pantothenic acid; these are all good for health and general wellbeing. It is also high in fibre. Celery is often said to be good for reducing blood pressure; this may be due to its potassium content and the presence of phthalides, compounds that relax muscles around arteries.

A study by the University of Maryland Medical Center stated that 'eating celery could possibly reduce the risk of gastritis (inflammation of the stomach lining) because the vegetable's flavonoids may help stop the growth of unwanted gut bacteria that causes inflammation.'

100g Celery nutrition information
Calories 16, Sugar 1.8g, Iron 1%, Vitamin C 5%

Yin and Yang score
Yin +++++ Yang +++

Relation to Organs
Lungs, Spleen, Digestive System, Heart, Kidneys and Bones

CHINESE CABBAGE

There are two groups of Chinese leaf vegetables often used in Chinese cuisine: the *Pekinensis Group* (napa cabbage) and the *Chinensis Group* (bok choi).

In China, people have Chinese cabbage every day. There is an old Chinese saying, 'If you don't eat cabbage for 3 days, your eyes will burn and hurt (三天不吃青，双眼冒金星). It is one of the most common and healthiest leaf vegetables. It is very filling and good for curbing hunger pangs, making you feel full easily. It really is one of the finest vegetables for weight loss and wellbeing.

In Traditional Chinese medicine

Chinese cabbage has a high level of Yin energy (Qi). It is a neutral vegetable as it is neither sweet nor sour, nor is it cold or warm. It is beneficial for the spleen, liver, kidneys, lungs and heart, and nourishment of Qi and Yin.

- It helps the body's Yin energy; it tones dry skin and hairs caused by dehydration and toxic damage, eliminating toxins from the body heat system, so it is great if you suffer from skin disorders or are going through the menopause.
- It helps the lungs' Qi energy, increasing lung strength to bring oxygen into body. It helps the liver's Qi energy, regular flowing Qi, reducing stress and anxiety. It helps the spleen's Qi energy, converting digested food into valuable nutrients and removing water. It also helps the

kidneys by regularly flushing out toxins.
- It helps to digest fatty foods quickly so you can often see Chinese people eat fatty or meaty meals accompanied with Chinese cabbage.

It is one of best and most common vegetables, helping our bodies to heal after sickness or weakness, such as cold, flu, stomach or colon problems, or weakness of immune system, etc. The more you eat, the more health benefits you derive from the food.

Its primary health benefits are as below:

- Helping weight loss
- Helping reduce hunger
- Helping the body to detox
- Helping the immune system
- Helping anti-ageing
- Helping constipation

Chinese cabbage is an excellent source of vitamin C; in fact, it has a higher level of vitamin C, vitamin A and iron than most vegetables. Vitamin A is a fat soluble vitamin that is also a powerful antioxidant; it plays a critical role in maintaining healthy vision, neurological function, healthy skin, and more. Vitamin A – like all antioxidants – is involved in reducing inflammation through fighting free radical damage. Vitamin C, also known as ascorbic acid, is necessary for the growth, development and repair of all body tissues.

Chinese cabbage has a high potassium content; it helps

support healthy brain function, relieve hypertension and regulate blood sugar. It is an extremely important mineral if you want to stay on top of health.

100 gram Chinese cabbage nutrition information

Calories 13, Sugar 1.2g, Iron 4%, Vitamin C 75%, Vitamin A 89%

Yin and Yang score

Yin +++++ Yang ++

Relation to Organs

Lungs, Liver, Spleen, Digestive System, Kidneys and Heart

TOFU

Tofu is a Chinese name which means 'bean curd' and is derived from soya beans. It is made by curdling fresh soya milk, pressing it into a solid block and then cooling it. It can be liquid, soft, firm, or extra firm, dried or fresh. Tofu is the most popular food in the slimming world now. It has a long history dating back to Taoism and Chinese Buddhism and is used as 'meat' in the Taoist and Chinese Buddhist diet. Nowadays, it is one of the finest foods replacing animal fat in the diet of vegans and vegetarians.

In Traditional Chinese medicine

Tofu has a Yang energy source and a Yin energy source, providing nourishment for all organs in the body. It provides nourishment of Qi, blood, Yin and Yang. It helps the body to function and repair; it provides strength for the muscle, tissues and organs, providing energy that is required by the body growing and repairing muscles, bones, hair, blood, etc. It is easy to digest and has fewer toxins compared to other general food.

- It boosts the body's Yin energy, keeping the body calm, aiding relaxation, sleeping and concentration. It helps prevent memory loss, improves vision, and treats the symptoms of menopause, fatigue and weak bones.
- It boosts the body's Yang energy. It helps the lungs, in particular with helping to breath, bringing fresh oxygen into the blood and helping to exhale out toxic air. It is easy to digest and comfortable for the stomach and colon to process. It strengthens the heart and prevents damage. It helps the kidneys' Jing (a special hormone quality in the West and special blood essence in Traditional Chinese Medicine) level, preventing signs of ageing that causes loss of body strength. It is one of the best foods to help the body recover from sickness or weakness.
- It boosts the blood, increasing blood quality to help fertility function and memory.

Its primary health benefits are as below:

- Helping in loss weight
- Helping the immune system

- Helping boost energy
- Helping digestion

Lots of studies published show that tofu contains phytoestrogens called isoflavones. It is similar in structure to the female hormone oestrogen and it therefore mimics the action of oestrogen produced by the body. It can help women pre-menopause, during menopause or after menopause to replace oestrogen. It helps to reduce symptoms of hot flush, sweating and other common menopausal symptoms.

A study by The American Institute for Cancer Research (AICR) even stated that eating just 1-2 servings of soya foods could have the potential to lower breast cancer risk and for some cancer survivors, it can lower mortality and tumour recurrence rates.

100 gram Tofu nutrition information
Calories 76, Sugar 0%, Iron 30%, Calcium 35%, Vitamin C 0%

Yin and Yang score
Yin ++++ Yang ++++

Relation to Organs
Lungs, Liver, Spleen, Heart, Kidneys, Bones, Hair and Brain

BLACK MUSHROOM

Black mushroom is also commonly called sawtooth oak mushroom, black forest mushroom, golden oak mushroom and oakwood mushroom.

Black mushroom is regarded by both Taoists and Chinese herbalists as magic food, and features prominently in the Taoist and Buddhist diets as 'meat'. Nowadays, it often replaces animal fat in vegan and vegetarian diets. It not only provides you with major nutrition, but it also helps with cleaning up your internal system to keep it in the best condition. Apart from that, it can assist you in weight loss or to maintain a healthy lifestyle and keep you slim. It also has strong healing properties and medical qualities.

In Traditional Chinese Medicine

Black mushroom has a Yin energy source and a Yang energy source. It is tasteless and gel like, and is good for the nourishment of Qi, blood, Yin and Yang and the whole body system. It is the strongest Yang energy boosting food and also the best Yin energy maintaining food product.

- It helps with the regulation of Qi, allowing it to flow freely and preventing Qi blockage in the energy channel which can cause body pain, headache or chest pain. It helps the lungs' Qi flow, bringing fresh oxygen into the blood. It helps the spleen's Qi, regulating food digestion and helping to turn it into nutrition for the body. It also helps the kidneys' Qi, reducing water retention.

- It helps regulate Yang energy, and can be used to treat tiredness and fatigue. It increases Yin energy and blood level, helping body regeneration. It is one of best foods for anti-ageing and weight loss. Furthermore, it is good for detoxification. You can eat it as often as you like, in fact, the more you eat the better you feel.
- It nourishes the blood and Yin, and is excellent food for your brain function, heart and fertility function.

Throughout history, the black mushroom has been considered as one of best natural medicines to treat tumours or excessive body fat.

Its primary health benefits are as below:

- Helping weight loss
- Helping the immune system
- Helping in anti-ageing
- Helping body detoxification

Shiitake mushrooms can help improve the immune system. The Institute of Food and Agricultural Sciences also found that not only do black mushrooms enhance the immune system, they can also significantly reduce the inflammation that the immune system produces.

The shiitake mushroom has been found to help with weight loss. A 2011 study published in the *Journal of Obesity* examined the effects of shiitake mushrooms on fat dispositions, energy efficiency and body fat index, and found significant effects of dietary intervention on body weight gain.

Shiitake mushrooms help anaemia caused by reduced vitamin B6 levels; because shiitake mushrooms contain 15% vitamin B as well as vitamin B6, it improves metabolism helping the body convert food into energy.

100g Fresh black mushroom (Fresh shiitake mushroom) nutrition information

Calories 34, Sugar 2.4g, Iron 2%, Vitamin C 0%, Vitamin B-6 15%

Yin and Yang score

Yin +++++ Yang ++++

Relation to Organs

Lungs, Liver, Spleen, Heart, Kidneys, Bones, Hair and Brains

BLACK FUNGUS

The scientific name of black fungus is auricularia polytricha. It also called wood ear fungus, wood fungus, ear fungus and cloud fungus.

It grows above the ground of some humid climates, living with old trees or deadly wood in the shade, such as pacific islands, or forest, or high mountains. It has been traditionally used for food as well as medicine, and often replaces meat in the diets of vegans and vegetarians in China.

In Traditional Chinese medicine

It has both a Yang and a Yin energy source. It is tasteless and gel-like and benefits Qi, blood, Yin and Yang, and all bodily functions. It helps build body muscles and provides nourishment for the bones, blood, hair etc. It provides strength for the body. It gives the lungs' strength, improving Qi exchanged with natural earth, flowing it into the blood.

- It gives the heart strength, improving heart Qi, ensuring it flows easily, thereby reducing the chance of clots.
- It gives the kidneys' strength, improving kidney Qi, removing toxins and keeping the body in good condition. It protects the body from liver damage due to its detoxing ability. It helps the spleen's Qi, regulating food digestion progress and carrying out waste. It is a calming and relaxing food product for the body, keeping the body in smooth working order.
- It helps the blood, improving the quality, particularly special for the brain, heart, kidneys and fertility function.
- It helps the body's Yin, nourishing and strengthening the body, joints, ligaments and skin collagen.
- It helps the body's Yang, powerful in prolonging energy and the function of fertility, memory and the heart.

Additionally, I would like to mention that the black fungus is the best protector for our bodies, as its gel like texture acts like a sea sponge and keeps the body system clean. It is thought to be rich in anti-ageing and detoxing properties.

Its primary health benefits are as below:

- Helping in weight loss
- Helping our immune system
- Helping the body to detoxify
- Helping with anti-ageing

A recent study by the Mycological Society of San Francisco found that black fungus has a chemical that inhibits blood clotting. It is a special plant for anti-clotting, anti-thrombosis, reducing blood fat, lowering blood viscosity, softening the blood vessel and ensuring that the blood flows smoothly.

Black fungus contains a higher level of iron compared to other vegetables. When eaten regularly, it can enrich blood and prevent iron deficiency (anaemia). It also contains high levels of calcium and protein.

It contains rich dietary fibres, and is particularly good for promoting movement of the stomach and intestine to help digestion, using its fibre to remove toxins (especially if you've had a meal with wine).

100 gram Dried black fungus nutrition information (10-15 medium-sized pieces)

Calories 200, Sugar 0%, Iron 33%, Vitamin C 0%, Vitamin A 0%, Dietary Fibre 28%, Calcium 16%, Protein (9.3g) 19%

Yin and Yang score

Yin +++++Yang ++++

Relation to Organs

Lungs, Liver, Spleen, Heart, Kidneys, Bones, Hair and Brain

Other vegetables that are good for weight loss

- Asparagus
- Beansprouts
- Bell peppers
- Bok choi
- Broccoli
- Carrot
- Cauliflower
- Green Beans
- Greens
- Leeks
- Lettuce
- Onion
- Spinach
- Spring Onion
- Snow beans
- Sweetcorn
- Tomatoes
- Yellow Squash

CHAPTER 7

Guidance and Weight Loss Recipes

Daily path to weight loss –
A.B.C.D Rotation

Life is busy in modern days and it is not the same as it was 3,000 years ago. Many of us are facing challenges just trying to manage our daily lives through normal routine. However, the Chinese are still practicing their ancient life routine during each meal time, known as the A.B.C.D table. The A.B.C.D rotation consists of drinking tea, having meals, exercising and eating fruits. The Chinese believe this rotation will help the body to get the energy it needs by injecting new energy.

From a quality and quantity perspective, the A.B.C.D routine should be customised for each individual. What's more, the needs of the individual changes day by day, and it depends on the balance of Yin and Yang of

143

your body on each particular day. In the morning, your body needs Yang and Qi energy in preparation for the whole day's work. When you follow a good breakfast routine, such as having fruit and tea and also good food, your body will be supplied with the maximum amount of Yang and Qi energy.

By lunchtime, the level of Yang and Qi energy in our body has been reduced gradually after 4 or 5 hours work. We will need to replenish this energy to fuel the rest of the day, and our body also needs Yin energy to maintain the flow of blood around the body allowing it to function normally.

At lunch, our intake of food, liquid and fruit combined with exercise depends on the requirements of the body. In addition, in China, people will have a siesta (nap) between 15 and 60 minutes after lunch, if it is possible.

After a long day, evening is the time for us to rest. We will need to reduce the level of Yang and Qi energy to the minimum we need. Furthermore, we should also switch off our mind and relax our body to get ourselves ready for a good night's sleep.

Occasionally, social events can throw our healthy routine away, such as meeting up with friends, special events and holidays. We could end up eating and drinking insensibly. However, please don't let those occasional social events worry you. Our body weight or general health cannot be changed by one meal or one day of activities as long as we drink more detoxing tea and eat less the following day. Our body will be balanced again. Remember, one meal or one day's over eating will not cause you to gain weight. But if you don't follow the A.B.C.D rotation, you will gain weight.

The A.B.C.D rotation consist of: Drinks, Exercise, Meal (see Recipes) and Fruits:

A. DRINKING

1. Cold Drinks

Cold water – a glass of cold tap water

Carrot water – 3-5 slices of fresh carrot in a glass of cold water

Cucumber water – 1-2 slices of fresh cucumber in a glass of cold water

Ginger water – 2-3 slices of fresh ginger in a glass of cold water

Lemon water – 2-3 slices of fresh lemon in a glass of cold water

Mint water – 1-2 sprigs of fresh mint leaves (or however many you prefer) in a glass of cold water

2. Hot Drinks

Lemon tea – 2-3 slices of fresh lemon in a cup of hot water

Mint tea – Fresh mint leaves (to taste) in a cup of hot water

Ginger tea – 2-3 slices of fresh ginger in a cup of hot water

Camomile Tea – 1 camomile tea bag in a cup of boiling water

3. Chinese Tea

Green Tea – Use 3g dry green tea leaves with 500ml
nearly boiled water

Wu-long Tea – Use 3g dry wu-long tea leaves with
500ml nearly boiled water

Jasmine Tea – Use 3g dry jasmine tea leaves with 500ml
nearly boiled water

Long Jing Tea – Use 3g dry long jing tea leaves with
500ml nearly boiled water

B. MEAL (SEE RECIPES)

C. FRUITS

After each meal, you can eat one or a mixture of fruits,
as a portion akin to 1-2 apples.

Apple – 1-2 after each meal

Melon – 2-3 pieces after each meal

Pineapple – 2-3 pieces after each meal

Kiwi – 1-2 after each meal

Peaches – 1-2 after each meal

Oranges – 1-2 after each meal

Strawberries – 10-15 after each meal

Pear – 1-2 after each meal

D. EXERCISE

Time – 15-45 minutes depending on your schedule
There are two types of exercise, one that is intensive and
makes you sweat as well as increases your heart rate, the
other that is more relaxing. The type needed depends on
the time of day.

Type of Exercise

Running

Fast walking

Chinese martial arts, such as Thai Ji Quang (太极拳) or
Qi Gong (气功)

Group dancing

Gym, Swimming

Cycling

Stretching

Etc.

Morning rotation: Drink, Exercise, Breakfast and Fruit.

Lunch rotation: Drink, Lunch, Fruit and Exercise.

Evening rotation: Drink, Evening meal, Fruit and Exercise.

General daily practice guidelines

Many people are fascinated by Chinese recipes, the combination of ingredients, and the different food used in each meal. How and why do we select these ingredients and cook these foods to eat?

Here are some examples of the role Yin and Yang balance plays in each Chinese recipe and each meal:

Colour: On one plate, we seldom use vegetables of the same colour. We combine red, white, green, black or red, dark and light colours.

Ingredients: We choose vegetables with meat or fish,

and never mix meat and fish. E.g. seafood is Yin and meat is Yang; vegetables are Yin and seafood is Yang. Tofu is Yin and meat is Yang; vegetables are Yin and black mushrooms are Yang.

Source of flavour: such as salt to sugar, vinegar to sugar, spicy to salty, soy bean sauce to salt etc. This can often change the recipe due to the Yin and Yang balance, e.g. Chinese often add vinegar or wine into cooking, or add spicy chilli.

Food texture: such as soft to hard, where the soft ingredient will be Yin and easily digestible, and the hard ingredient will be Yang and harder to digest. Likewise, liquid food is Yin and easily digested, whereas firm food is Yang and needs time to digest. Leafy vegetables are Yin as they are easily digested, but beans and nuts are Yang as they easily process gas and need more time to digest.

Combinations in each meal: In one meal, Chinese people will make sure they have solid food, animal fat (Yang), vegetables and soup (Yin).

A guide to the Yin Yang recipes

MEASURES

Measures

tsp = teaspoon
tbsp = tablespoon
1 slice ginger = 1g
1/2 onion = 5g
1 tsp garlic, finely chopped = 5g

1/2 tsp salt = 1g
1 tbsp olive or sunflower oil = 6g
1 tsp wine (red or white) = 3g
1 tsp light soy sauce = 3g
1 tbsp light soy sauce = 7g
1 tsp chilli bean sauce = 3g
1 tbsp chilli bean sauce = 7g
1 tsp salted black bean with ginger = 3g
1 tbsp salted black bean with ginger = 6g
1 tbsp water = 6g
1 tbsp mixed salted bean = 7g
1 tbsp dry beans or dry nuts = 10g
1 tbsp dry fruits = 5g
1 tbsp rice =10g
1 cup water = 240g

Dice: cut into smaller pieces, can also be used to cut vegetables into cubes

Chop: cut into larger pieces, less precise

Mince: dice into as small a piece as possible

Strips: a French cooking term, also referred as julienne; cut about 3 inches long and 1/16 to 1/8 inch thick.

Large chop: double the size of a £2 coin

Medium chop: size of a £2 coin

Small chop: half of a £2 coin

COMMON INGREDIENTS AND TECHNIQUES

Wok: easily bought in a shop or online

Electric rice cooker/steamer: easily bought in a shop or online

Rice: preferably Chinese, Indian, Thai

Vinegar: cider apple vinegar

Wine: 13-20% red or white wine

Oil: sunflower oil or olive oil

Dried black mushroom or dry black fungus: Soak it in warm water for at least 3 hours.

Dried fruits: Put into a bowl of warm water for 60 minutes

Dry seeds or dry nuts: Put into a bowl of warm water for 12 hours

When you make Chinese rice porridge, use 1 part rice to 6 parts water

You can find the ingredients for these recipes in health food shops, oriental supermarkets or Chinese clinics

Microwave on Auto settings, using a ceramic plate covered with cling film

Oven temperature: set to 150°C (unless otherwise stated)

Use kitchen foil that is 2 1/2 times the size of the vegetable/meat/fish you are cooking so that you can fold it over to create a parcel when cooking

Enjoy making these recipes and use your creativity and imagination to gain experience over time.

General role of cooking

1. Flavour: ginger, spring onion, coriander
   - Add ginger and spring onion before animal meat. When we cook animal fat (fish, seafood, pork, beef...), we need first to put the oil on maximum heat, stir for few seconds, then add ginger and spring onions, stirring for a few seconds, and then add animal fat.
   - Add spring onion and coriander before serving.

2. Texture: soft, medium, hard
   - Soft texture needed for all leaf vegetables such as spinach, Chinese leaf, tomatoes, seaweed, tofu, etc. Cook them for between 3-5 minutes.
   - Medium texture needed for vegetables cut into thin pieces (such as courgette, aubergine, cucumber and white broccoli) or chopped vegetables such as bell pepper, celery root, white radish, etc. Cook them for between 8-15 minutes.
   - Hard texture needed for vegetables cut into large pieces, such as white radish, runner beans, asparagus, bell pepper, green peas and beans, dried black fungus, and dried black mushroom. There are two ways to cook: one is boiling them for 5-10 minutes, then rinsing them under a tap with cold water, then mixing them together with other vegetables; the other way is to cook them for 15-25 minutes on a medium heat and cook slowly, adding a little water to prevent drying or burning.

151

3. Sauce or flavour in powder form etc.

Animal meat has a strong taste so we add wine, vinegar, special sauces or ingredients in powder form.

- We can always mix wine and vinegar with animal fat in a bowl for a few minutes before cooking, or cook animal fat 5-10 minutes before everthing else is ready.
- Or you can add wine or vinegar a few minutes after cooking the meat. For special sauces and ingredients in powder form, it is normal to stir into the cooking 5-10 minutes before the end.

4. Animal fat

- If they are small dices or thin pieces, you should stir for 5-10 minutes until cooked.
- If they are large dices or pieces, you should first stir on a maximum heat for a few minutes, then turn the heat down to medium/low medium and slowly cook for 15-25 minutes.
- For animal fat with different textures: animal fat with a hard texture will always take longer to cook than others.

Breakfast weight loss recipes

CHINESE RICE PORRIDGES (ZHOU)

- Portion: 1-2 people
- Preparation time: 25-30 minutes
- Rice porridge is very flexible. You can use a combination any of the following: any nuts, seeds, dry fruits, fresh seafood, meat or vegetables to mix with steamed rice (the softer the better). You can eat rice porridge with a little salt or honey according to your taste. The common Chinese way to serve Chinese rice porridge is to accompany it with pickled vegetables, such as cucumber, white radish, cabbage, ginger or garlic as side dishes, similar to olives in the West. Also, when you eat Chinese rice porridge, it can be accompanied with a hard-boiled egg or you can steam ready-made dim sum. If you only eat Chinese porridge, you may still feel hungry due to it being easily digested.

How to make Chinese Rice Porridge
Using a saucepan

1. Put a combination of nuts, seeds, vegetables, meat or seafood into a saucepan of water, take to the boil (about 5 minutes)
2. Turn down the heat and simmer for 25 minutes.

3. Add the steamed rice, mix and simmer for a further 5 minutes.

4. It is ready to serve.

Using a digital rice cooker

1. Put a combination of any nuts, seeds, vegetables, meat or seafood into a saucepan of water, take to the boil (about 25 minutes), then add steamed rice for 5 minutes more.

GOJI BERRIES RICE PORRIDGE

Ingredients:
90g steamed rice
2 tbsp (10g) dried goji berries
2 tbsp (20g) dried black eyed beans
2 tbsp (20g) dried chana dal
2 cups (500ml) water

Method:
1. Wash and soak the chana dal and black eyed beans in a bowl of cold water for 12 hours. Wash and soak the dried goji berries in a bowl for 10 minutes.

2. Put the chana dal and black eyed beans into fresh water into a digital rice cooker and cook for 25 minutes. After the 25 minutes, add the steamed rice and goji berries for 5 minutes then remove.

3. It is ready to serve.

Alternatively you can use a saucepan

100g Goji berries nutrition information

Calories 90, Fat 0.4g, Sugar 3g, Iron 6%

Yin and Yang Score

Yang ++++ Yin ++++

Relation to Organs

Liver, Kidneys, Spleen, Heart and Lungs

SWEETCORN RICE PORRIDGE

Ingredients:
90g steamed rice
2 tbsp (20g) fresh sweet corn
2 tbsp (20g) fresh garden peas
1/3 tsp salt
2 cups (500ml) water

Method:
1. Wash the peas. Cut the corn from the sweet corn cob.

2. Put the sweet corn, garden peas and salt together with water into a digital rice cooker for 25 minutes. Then add the steamed rice for 5 minutes.

3. It is ready to serve.

Alternatively you can use a saucepan

100g Sweet corn nutrition information
Calories 111, Fat 1.2g, Sugar 3.2g, Iron 2 %

Yin and Yang Score
Yang + Yin ++++

Relation to Organs
Spleen, Kidneys, Sexual function, Liver, Heart and Lungs

MIXED BEAN RICE PORRIDGE

Ingredients:
90g steamed rice
2 tbsp (20g) dried black eyed beans
2 tbsp (20g) dried kidney beans
1 tbsp (10g) dried pistachio kernels
1 tbsp (10g) dried pecans
2 cups (500ml) water

Method:
1. Soak the red beans, kidney beans, pistachio kernels and pecans in cold water for 12 hours.

2. Put all the beans and nuts with the water into a digital rice cooker and cook for 25 minutes. Then add the steamed rice for a further 5 minutes.

3. It is ready to serve.

Alternatively you can use a saucepan

100g Kidney beans nutrition information
Calories 127, Fat 0.5g, Sugar 0.32g, Iron 12%

Yin and Yang Score
Yang ++ Yin ++++

Relation to Organs
Lungs, Liver, Heart and Kidneys

SHIITAKE MUSHROOM RICE PORRIDGE

Ingredients
90g steamed rice
3 fresh or dried shiitake (black) mushrooms
10g roasted almonds
1/2 tbsp sunflower oil
1/3 tsp salt
20g celery leaves
2 cups (500ml) water

Method:
1. Chop the shiitake mushrooms and celery leaves into small pieces. Crush the roasted almond into small pieces.

2. Put the steamed rice, shiitake mushrooms, almonds, celery leaves, oil, salt and water into a digital rice cooker and cook for 8 minutes.

3. It is ready to serve.

Alternatively you can use a saucepan

100g Almond nutrition information
Calories 575, Fat 49g, Sugar 3.9g, Iron 20%

Yin and Yang Score
Yang +++++ Yin +

Relation to Organs
Kidneys, Heart, Liver, Spleen and Lungs

PRAWN PROTEIN RICE PORRIDGE

Ingredients:
90g steamed rice
3 tbsp (15g) king prawns
10g ginger
10g spring onion
1tbsp sunflower oil
1/3 tsp salt
2 cups (500ml) water

Method:
1. Cut the king prawns into small dices. Peel and chop the ginger into small pieces. Chop the spring onions.

2. Put the prawns, ginger, steamed rice, salt, oil and water into a digital rice cooker, and cook for 8 minutes.

3. Sprinkle the spring onion on top of the rice porridge before serving.

Alternatively you can use a saucepan

100g Ginger nutrition information
Calories 80, Fat 1g, Sugar 1.7g, Iron 3%

Yin and Yang score
Yang +++ Yin +

Relation to Organs
Heart, Lungs, Liver, Kidneys and Spleen

CHICKEN RICE PORRIDGE

Ingredients:
90g steamed rice
30g fresh chicken breast
10g ginger
5g spring onions
1/2 tsp white wine
1/3 tsp salt
2 cups (500ml) water

Method:
1. Cut the chicken breast into small pieces, then mix with white wine in a bowl for a few minutes. Peel and chop the ginger. Chop the spring onions.

2. Put the chicken breast pieces, ginger, salt, steamed rice and water into a digital rice cooker, and cook for 8 minutes.

3. Sprinkle the spring onion on top of the rice porridge before serving.

Alternatively you can use a saucepan

100g Spring onion nutrition information
Calories 4, Fat 0.1g, Sugar 4.2g, Iron 1%

Yin and Yang Score
Yang + Yin +

Relation to Organs
Spleen, Kidneys and Heart

PORK RICE PORRIDGE

Ingredients:
90g steamed rice
25g lean pork
2 shiitake mushrooms
1 tsp red wine
1/3 salt
5g spring onions
2 cups (500ml) water

Method:
1. Dice the pork then marinate with the wine in a bowl for few minutes. Chop the shiitake mushrooms. Peel and chop the ginger. Chop the spring onions.

2. Put the pork pieces, ginger, shiitake mushrooms, steamed rice and water together into a digital rice cooker, and cook for 20 minutes.

3. Sprinkle the spring onion on top of the rice porridge before serving.

Alternatively you can use a saucepan but cook for 30 minutes.

100g Black mushroom nutrition information
Calories 34, Fat 0.5g, Sugar 2.4g, Iron 2%

Yin and Yang Score
Yang +++++ Yin +++++

Relation to Organs
Lungs, Kidneys and Liver

Egg Recipes

- Serving: All recipes serve 1
- Preparation time: 5-10 minutes
- Eggs are fat free, good for boosting energy and packed with fibre.

SLICED EGGS WITH CUCUMBER

Ingredients:

2 hard-boiled eggs

1/2 peeled cucumber

1/2 peeled carrot

A little table salt

A little olive or sesame oil

1 tsp premium light soy sauce

Method:

1. Peel and thinly slice at an angle the cucumber and carrot. Hard boil the eggs and slice.
2. Lay the sliced eggs, cucumber and carrot on three separate parts of the plate.
3. Mix the oil, salt and light soy sauce together, then pour over the cucumber and carrot before serving.

100g Cucumber nutrition information

Calories 16, Fat 0.1g, Sugar 1.7g, Iron 1%

Yin and Yang Score

Yang ++ Yin +++++

POACHED EGGS WITH TOMATO

Ingredients
2 eggs
2 medium sized tomatoes
5g spring onion
pinch of salt
500ml (2 cups) boiling water

Method
1. Slice the tomatoes. Chop the spring onion.

2. Place a pan of boiling water on a low to medium heat. Break the eggs into a bowl, then carefully pour them into the water and cover the pan. Cook for about 5 minutes then remove the cover and turn off the heat. Using a perforated spoon, carefully remove the eggs to a plate, taking care not to break the yolks.

3. Lay the tomato slices on the side of the plate.

4. Decorate with the spring onion pieces and add salt to taste before serving.

100g Tomatoes nutrition information
Calories 18, Fat 0.2g, Sugar 2.6g, Iron 1%

Yin and Yang Score
Yang +++ Yin +++++

STIR-STEAM EGGS

Ingredients:
1 egg (at room temperature)
40g red bell pepper
60g celery
1 tbsp water
1/3 tsp salt
1/3 tsp ground black pepper
1tsp sesame oil

Method

1. Slice the red bell pepper and celery at an angle.

2. Put a non-stick frying pan on a medium to high heat. Break the egg into a small bowl and quickly put it in the middle of the pan. Turn the heat to low-medium and cook uncovered for one minute until the egg has started to turn white. Pour water around the edge of the egg, cover the pan for one minute or more then turn off the heat (the yolk should still be soft). Transfer the egg to a plate.

3. Place the raw sliced celery and red bell pepper to the side of the egg.

4. Mix the salt and oil then pour over the pepper and celery.

5. Sprinkle a little ground black pepper to your taste before serving.

100g Red bell pepper nutrition information

Calories 31, Fat 0.3g, Sugar 4.2g, Iron 2%

Yin and Yang Score

Yang ++ Yin ++++

All egg recipes can be served for lunch or as an evening meal

Stir-fried rice recipes

- Portion: 2-3 persons
- Preparation time: 10-15 minutes
- Rice must be steamed first then cooled for 30 minutes before using

FRIED RICE AND TOFU

Ingredients
1 (280g) bowl of rice
60g firm tofu
2 dry black fungus
40g red bell pepper
30g white broccoli florets
70g green broccoli florets
20g spring onion
2 tbsp olive oil
1/2 tsp salt

Method
1. Chop the tofu, red bell pepper and white and green broccoli florets into medium pieces. Soak the dried black fungus, rinse and chop. Cut the spring onion into strips.
2. Put a wok on a high heat, add oil for a few seconds then add the tofu, broccoli florets, red bell pepper and black fungus. Stir for 10 minutes then add rice and salt, and stir for 10 more minutes. In the meantime,

add 1-2 tbsp water to prevent dryness or burning.
3. Add spring onion before serving.

100g White broccoli nutrition information
Calories 34, Fat 0.37g, Sugar 1.7g, Iron 4%

Yin and Yang Score
Yang ++ Yin ++++

FRIED RICE AND SHRIMPS

Ingredients
1 (280g) bowl of rice
50g fresh peeled shrimps
1 egg
30g carrots
60g garden peas
20g spring onion
2 tbsp olive oil
1/2 tsp salt
1 tsp light soy sauce
2 tbsp cold water

Method
1. Chop the carrots and spring onion into medium pieces.

2. Put a wok on a high heat, add oil for a few seconds then add the carrot and fresh garden peas. Stir for 5 minutes then add the rice and continue to stir for 10 minutes. Add the shrimps, salt and light soy sauce for a further 5 minutes. Add a little water as necessary. Then adds spring onion a few seconds.

3. It is ready to serve.

100g Garden peas nutrition information
Calories 81, Fat 0.4g, Sugar 5.67g, Iron 8%

Yin and Yang Score
Yang +++ Yin ++++

FRIED RICE AND CHICKEN BREAST

Ingredients:
1(280g) bowl of rice
50g chicken breast
2 dried black mushrooms
40g red bell pepper
40g green bell pepper
2 asparagus
30g ginger
20g spring onion
2 tbsp olive oil
1/2 tsp salt
1/2 tsp white wine
1 tsp light soy sauce
2 tbsp water

Method:
1. Chop the red bell pepper, green bell pepper, asparagus, spring onion and chicken breast into medium sized pieces. Peel and chop the ginger. Soak the dried black mushroom and chop.

2. Put a wok on a medium high heat, add oil for a few seconds then add the ginger, chicken and wine for 5 minutes. Transfer to a bowl, keeping the oil in the wok. Then add all the vegetables and black mushroom back into the wok, and stir for 10 minutes. Then add the rice and cooked chicken back into the wok and continue to stir for 10 minutes. Add the salt, light soy sauce and stir for 3 more

minutes. Add water if necessary to prevent burning or drying out.

3. It is ready to serve.

100g Green bell pepper nutrition information
Calories 26, Fat 0.2g, Sugar 2.4g, Iron 1%

Yin and Yang Score
Yang + Yin ++++

With the stir fried rice recipes, you can add more vegetables or eggs as you wish. These can also be served for lunch or as an evening meal

Liquid food recipes

- Portion: 1-2 people
- Preparation time: 5-10 minutes
- Beans and nuts are considered 'meat' quality foods for vegetarians or vegans. They are high in Yang energy. Fruits and vegetables are high in Yin energy
- You can make the drinks by using a blender or liquidiser

MIXED DRY NUTS

Ingredients
10g dry pecans
10 dry almonds
10g dry blanched peanuts
30g dry kidney beans
Water
All nuts and beans:water = 1:4 (tbsp)

Method
1. Soak the dry nuts and beans for 12 hours.
2. Put them into a blender and follow instructions. Sieve into a cup and put in the microwave for 1 minute.

100g Pecan nutrition information
Calories 690, Fat 72g, Sugar 4g, Iron 13%

Yin and Yang Score
Yang +++++ Yin +

MIXED WALNUTS

Ingredients
20g dry walnuts
10 g dry pine nuts
30g black eyed beans
10g dry raw cashews
Water
All nuts:water = 1:5 (tbsp)

Method
1. Soak the dry nuts and beans for 12 hours.

2. Put them into a blender and follow instructions. Sieve into a cup and put in the microwave for 1 minute.

100g Walnut nutrition information
Calories 654, Fat 65g, Sugar 2.6g, Iron 10%

Yin and Yang Score
Yang +++++ Yin +

MIXED FRESH FRUIT JUICE

Ingredients:
30g apple
30g water melon
30g kiwi
30g Orange
30g Strawberry

Method
1. Peel and chop the kiwi fruit. Cut the skin off the watermelon and orange, and chop. Chop the apple and strawberries.

2. Put in a blender, sieve and serve.

100g Kiwi nutrition information
Calories 61, Fat 0.52g, Sugar 9g, Iron 2%

Yin and Yang Score
Yang ++++ Yin +++++

VEGETABLE DRINK

Ingredients
30g cucumber
30g carrot
30g celery
20g kale
Water
All vegetables:water = 1:3

Method
1. Chop all vegetables.

2. Put in a blender, sieve and serve.

100g Kale nutrition information
Calories 16, Fat 0.2g, Sugar 1.8g, Iron 1%

Yin and Yang Score
Yang ++++ Yin +++++

You can try making different types of drinks by adding different nuts, beans, fruits and vegetables

LUNCH WEIGHT LOSS RECIPES

SOUP

- Serving: 2-3 people
- Preparation time: 10-15 minutes

TOFU AND CHINESE CABBAGE SOUP

Ingredients
80g tofu
40g Chinese cabbage leaf
1/2 carrot
5g ginger
5g spring onion
1/2 tsp salt
1 tbsp olive oil
2 cups (500ml) boiling water

Method

1. Dice the tofu. Peel and slice the carrot and ginger. Cut the spring onion into small pieces. Slice the Chinese cabbage at an angle.

2. Put a pan of boiling water on a medium heat, add the Chinese cabbage, carrot, ginger, salt and olive oil, and simmer for 10 minutes. Add the tofu and cook for 3 minutes, then add the spring onion and salt for a few seconds.

3. It is ready to serve.

100g Chinese cabbage nutrition information
Calories 13, Fat 0.2g, Sugar 1.2g, Iron 4%

Yin and Yang Score
Yang ++ Yin ++++++

TOFU AND HAI DAI (海带)
SEAWEED SOUP

Ingredients:
80g tofu
3g dry seaweed
3g coriander
1 tbsp olive oil
1/2 tsp salt
2 cups (500ml) boiling water

Method

1. Cut the tofu into strips. Cut the coriander into small pieces.

2. Put a pan of boiling water on a medium heat, add the tofu and olive oil, and simmer for 5 minutes. Then add the seaweed, coriander and salt together for a few seconds, and stir them into the soup.

3. It is ready to serve.

100g Seaweed nutrition information

Calories 43, Fat 0.6g, Sugar 0.6g, Iron 16%

Yin and Yang Score

Yang ++++ Yin +++++

WHITE RADISH AND EXOTIC MUSHROOM SOUP

Ingredients:
150g white radish
30g fresh exotic mushroom
10g spring onion
5g fresh ginger
1 tbsp olive oil
1/2 tsp salt
1 tsp light soy sauce
2 cups (500ml) boiling water

Method:
1. Peel and cut the white radish into thin strips. Cut the exotic mushroom into thin strips. Cut the spring onion into small pieces. Peel and dice the ginger.

2. Put a pan of boiling water on a medium heat, add the white radish, fresh exotic mushroom, ginger and olive oil and simmer for 8 minutes. Then add the spring onion, salt and light soy sauce for a few seconds.

3. It is ready to serve.

100g White radish nutrition information
Calories 18, Fat 0.1g, Sugar 2.5g, Iron 2%

Yin and Yang Score
Yang +++ Yin +++++

SPINACH SOUP

Ingredients
10g baby spinach leaf
30g Shimeji mushrooms
10g carrots
10g ginger
1 tbsp olive oil
1/2 tsp salt
2 cups (500ml) boiling water

Method
1. Slice the shimeji mushrooms. Peel and slice the carrot and ginger.

2. Put a pan of boiling water on a medium heat then add the shimeji mushroom, carrot, ginger and olive oil. Simmer for 8 minutes then add the spinach and salt for a few seconds.

3. It is ready to serve.

100g Spinach nutrition information
Calories 18, Fat 0.1g, Sugar 2.5g, Iron 25%

Yin and Yang Score
Yang ++ Yin +++++

PORK SOUP

Method:
80g lean organic pork
3 dried black mushrooms
1 white radish
10g ginger
10g sparing onion
1 tbsp olive oil
1/2 tsp wine
1/2 tsp salt
2 cups (500ml) boiling water

Method

1. Cut the lean pork into strips then mix with white wine in a bowl. Soak the dry black mushroom and cut into strips. Peel and slice the white radish. Peel and cut the ginger into thin pieces. Cut the spring onion into pieces.

2. Put a pan on a medium heat, add the lean pork and simmer for couple minutes, then use a spoon to take off the film from the surface of the water. Then add the black mushrooms, white radish, ginger and olive oil. Simmer for 10 minutes then add the spring onion and salt for a few seconds.

3. It is ready to serve.

100g Baby pak choi nutrition information
Calories 13, Fat 0.2g, Sugar 1.2g, Iron 4%

Yin and Yang Score
Yang ++ Yin +++++

BABY CORN SOUP

Ingredients:
3 baby corn cobs
20g carrot
5g seaweed
10g green garden peas
1tbsp olive oil
1/2 tsp salt
2 cups (500ml) water

Method
1. Chop the baby corn into pieces. Peel and dice the carrot.

2. Put a pan of boiling water on a medium heat then add the baby corn, carrot, green garden peas, ginger and olive oil. Simmer for 10 minutes then add the spring onion, seaweed and salt for a few seconds. In the meantime, use chopsticks to stir and separate the seaweed leaves into soup.

3. It is ready to serve.

100g Green garden peas nutrition information
Calories 81, Fat 0.4g, Sugar 6.67g, Iron 8%

Yin and Yang Score
Yang +++ Yin ++++

KALE AND ERYNGII MUSHROOM SOUP

(Eryngii mushroom = Korean king oyster mushroom)

Ingredients:
20g soft leaf kale
20g eryngii mushroom
10g carrots
5g ginger
1 tbsp olive oil
1/2 tsp salt
2 cups (500ml) water

Method:
1. Chop the kale and eryngii mushrooms into medium pieces. Peel and slice the carrot and ginger into pieces.

2. Put a pan of boiling water on a medium heat then add the kale, mushrooms, ginger and olive oil together. Simmer for 6 minutes then add salt and cook for a few seconds.

3. It is ready to serve.

100g Kale nutrition information
Calories 49, Fat 0.9g, Sugar 0g, Iron 8%

Yin and Yang Score
Yang +++ Yin +++++

All these soups can be served as an evening meal. The soup can be made using all different kinds of vegetables, meat and seafood

Vegan recipes

- Portion: 1-2 people
- Preparation time: 15-25 minutes
- Microwave time: 3-5 minutes
- Sir-fry time: 15-25 minutes
- When microwaving make sure the plate is microwave safe and use microwavable cling film.
- Be careful when removing the plate from the microwave, and be sure to remove the cling film with a fork or chopstick to release the heat.
- During cooking, add a little water if necessary to prevent drying out or burning.

SILK TOFU BAO

Ingredients:
300g silk tofu
2 dried black fungus, soaked for 3 hours
10g spring onion
10g red bell pepper
1 tbsp olive oil
1 tsp sesame oil
1/2 tsp salt
2 tbsp premium light soy sauce

Method
1. Pour water onto the silk tofu with very light pressure and rinse. Then lay it on a deep flat-bottomed plate

and use a sharp knife to slice half way through the tofu. Chop the spring onion and red bell pepper into small pieces. Soak the black fungus and chop it into small pieces. Sprinkle the vegetables onto the tofu.

2. Mix the olive oil, sesame oil, salt and premium light soy sauce together in a bowl. Pour them over the portion.

3. Cover the plate with cling film and microwave for 3 minutes, then serve.

100g Tofu nutrition information

Calories 76, Fat 4.8g, Sugar 0%, Iron 30%

Yin and Yang score

Yang ++++ Yin ++++

AUBERGINES

Ingredients:
1 (150g) aubergine
15g garlic
20g red bell pepper
5g coriander
1 tbsp olive oil
1 tsp sesame oil
1/2 tsp salt
2 tbsp premium light soy sauce

Method
1. Cut the aubergine in two then cross-cut the flesh 2/3rds deep and place on a deep flat-bottomed plate. Peel and crunch the garlic pieces. Cut the red bell pepper into thin strips. Chop the coriander.

2. Mix the garlic and coriander together then sprinkle on top of the aubergine, then add the red bell pepper on top of the portion. Mix the olive oil, sesame oil, salt and light soy sauce together and pour over the portion.

3. Cover the plate with cling film, microwave for 4 minutes and serve.

100g Aubergine nutrition information
Calories 25, Fat 0.2g, Sugar 3.5g, Iron 1%

Yin and Yang score
Yang ++ Yin ++++

GREAT GRUB CLUB

Ingredients:

3 endive

3 dried black fungus

15g garlic

20g red bell pepper

20g green bell pepper

5g coriander

1 tbsp olive oil

1 tsp sesame oil

1/2 tsp salt

1 tbsp oyster sauce

2 tsp premium light soy sauce

Method

1. Cut the endive into two pieces. Soak the dried black fungus then chop into pieces. Peel and cut the garlic into small pieces. Cut the red and green bell pepper into strips. Cut the coriander to strips.

2. Put a pan of nearly boiled water on the heat, add the endive for 1 minute then sieve it under the tap and rinse. Bring the endive onto a deep-bottomed plate. Then add all the vegetables and black fungus on the top of the endive.

3. Mix the olive oil, sesame oil, salt and oyster and premium light soy sauce together, then pour over the endive portion.

4. Cover the plate with cling film, microwave for 2
   minute and serve.

100g Endive nutritional information

Calorie 17, Fat 0.2g, Sugar 0.3g, Iron 4%

Yin and Yang score

Yang + Yin +++++

RUNNER BEAN AND
YELLOW PEPPER STIR-FRY

Ingredients:
80g runner beans
80g yellow bell pepper
80g mixed cauliflower & broccoli florets
80g chestnut mushrooms
3 black fungus
3 tbsp olive oil
1 tsp salt
1 tbsp light sauce
3 tbsp water

Method
1. Soak and cut the black fungus into strips. Cut the runner beans, yellow bell pepper and half the cauliflower & broccoli florets into strips. Slice the chestnut mushrooms.

2. Put a wok on a maximum heat, add oil for a few seconds then add the runner beans, yellow bell pepper, cauliflower & broccoli florets, black fungus and chestnut mushrooms together. Stir for 10 minutes then turn heat down to medium, add the salt and light soy sauce then stir for 10 more minutes. Add water if necessary to prevent dryness and burning.

3. It is ready to serve.

100g Runner bean nutrition information
Calories 27, Fat 0, Sugar 3g, Iron 0%

Yin and Yang score

Yang +++ Yin ++++

ASPARAGUS AND CARROT

Ingredients:
150g asparagus
50g carrots
9 dry black mushrooms
3 tbsp olive oil
1 tsp sesame oil
1 tsp salt
1 tbsp oyster sauce
1 tbsp light soy sauce
1 tbsp water

Method
1. Soak the dry black mushrooms with storks removed. Cut the asparagus with the end of the stork removed. Peel and cut the carrot into strips.

2. Add the asparagus and carrots to a pan of boiling water, simmer for 5 minutes, sieve under tap water then place them on a plate.

3. Put a wok on a maximum heat, add olive oil for a few seconds then add the mushrooms and stir for 5 minutes. Add the salt, light soy sauce, oyster sauce together and stir for a few seconds, then add water and turn the heat down low for 15 minutes.

4. Bring the black mushrooms with the sauce together onto the portion of vegetables.

5. Pour the sesame oil on the top of the portion and serve.

100g Asparagus nutrition information

Calories 20, Fat 0.1g, Sugar 1.9g, Iron 11%

Yin and Yang score

Yang +++++ Yin +++

FIRM TOFU AND SHIITAKE MUSHROOM

Ingredients:
200g firm tofu
50g shiitake mushroom
10g red chilli
10g ginger
20g spring onion
3 tbsp olive oil
1 tsp salt
1 tbsp light soy sauce
2 tbsp water

Method
1. Cut the firm tofu and spring onion into medium strips. Cut the shiitake mushroom and peeled ginger into slices. Cut the red chilli into rings.

2. Put a wok on a maximum high heat, add oil for a few seconds then add the ginger, chilli, shiitake mushrooms and tofu together. Stir for 5 minutes then turn the heat down to medium and add the salt, light soy sauce and water. Simmer for 5 minutes then add the spring onion for a few seconds.

3. It is ready to serve.

100g Red chilli nutrition information
Calories 40, Fat 0.44g, Sugar 5.30g, Iron 6%

Yin and Yang score
Yang +++ Yin +

COURGETTE AND BROWN TOFU GAN

Ingredients:
100g mild green padron pepper
80g courgette
100g brown tofu gan
10g ginger
3 tbsp olive oil
1 tsp salt
1 tbsp oyster sauce
1 tbsp light soy sauce
2 tbsp water

Method
1. Cut the brown tofu gan and courgette into medium square pieces. Remove seeds from the padron pepper and slice. Peel and slice the ginger. Cut the spring onions into strips.

2. Put a wok on a maximum heat, add oil for a few seconds then add the ginger, courgette, padron pepper and tofu gan together. Stir for 10 minutes then turn the heat down to medium and add the salt, premium light soy sauce, oyster sauce and water. Stir for a further 10 minutes.

3. It is ready to serve.

100g Courgette nutrition information
Calories 17%, Fat 0.3g, Sugar 2.50g, Iron 2%

Yin and Yang score

Yang + Yin +++++

All of these recipes can also be served as an evening meal

Seafood recipes

- Portion: 2 people
- Preparation time: 15-30 minutes
- During cooking, add a little water if necessary to prevent drying out or burning.

VILLAGE FISH

Ingredients:
2 pieces of sea bass fillet
80g red onion
6 dried black fungus
10g ginger
10g coriander
3 tbsp sunflower oil
1/2 tsp salt
3 tbsp seasoned soy sauce for seafood
1 tsp cider apple vinegar
1 tsp white wine
3 tbsp water

Method
1. Cut the red onion into medium pieces. Peel and chop the ginger into medium pieces. Soak and chop the dried black fungus into medium pieces. Chop the coriander into strips. Cut the sea bass fillet into large pieces, then marinate with wine and vinegar in a bowl.

2. Put a wok on a maximum heat, add olive oil for a few seconds then add ginger and onion for a few seconds. Add the sea bass fillets and cook for 5 minutes. In the meantime, slowly stir to keep each piece complete then transfer everything to a bowl.

3. Put the wok back on the heat, add sunflower oil for a few seconds then add the black fungus and red onion together. Stir for 5 minutes then add the cooked sea bass fillet, salt, seasoned soy sauce for seafood and carefully stir slowly for 5 minutes. Add a little water if necessary.

4. Bring everything together on one plate, sprinkle coriander on top of the portion and serve.

100g Sea bass nutrition information
Calories 100, Fat 9g, Sugar 0.11g , Iron 2%

Yin and Yang score
Yang ++++ Yin ++++

ROMANTIC COD

Ingredients:
200g cod loins
8 red baby tomatoes
6 fresh shiitake mushrooms
10g spring onion
2 tbsp olive oil
1/2 tsp salt
3 tbsp seasoned soy sauce for seafood
1tsp white wine

Method
1. Cut the cod loins into square pieces then mix with wine in a bowl. Slice the shiitake mushrooms. Cut the baby tomatoes cross 3/4 deep, like an open flower. Chop the spring onion.

2. Using a deep flat-bottomed plate, lay the cod loin pieces and shiitake mushroom on opposite sides of the plate. Add the baby tomatoes in the middle on top.

3. Mix the oil, salt and seasoned soy sauce for seafood together then pour the sauce on the top of the portion. Cover the plate with cling film and microwave for 4 minutes.

4. Sprinkle the spring onion on to the portion before serving.

100g Cod loin nutrition information
Calorie 82, Fat 0.67g, Sugar 0, Iron 2%

Yin and Yang score
Yang ++++ Yin ++

DISNEY BEAUTY

Ingredients:
150g peeled Atlantic prawns
80g mini cos lettuce leaves
10g dried black fungus
10g ginger
5g coriander
2 tbsp olive oil
1tsp white wine
2 tbsp seasoned soy sauce for seafood

Method
1. Mix the Atlantic peeled prawns with wine in a bowl. Pull the mini cos lettuce leaves into separate pieces. Soak and cut the dried black fungus into large pieces. Cut the coriander into small pieces. Peel and cut the ginger into small pieces.

2. Using a deep flat-bottomed plate, lay the lettuce leaf pieces on the plate, place the peeled prawns on top then lay the black fungus around the prawns.

3. Mix the chopped ginger, coriander, salt, seasoned soy sauce for seafood and oil together, then pour them on top of the portion.

4. Cover with cling film then microwave for 3 minutes.

5. Sprinkle coriander on the portion before serving.

100g Peeled Atlantic prawns nutrition information
Calories 85, Fat 1.1g, Sugar 0.1g, Iron 0%

Yin and Yang score
Yang ++++ Yin ++

OLD BEAUTY

Ingredients:
200g scallops
1/2 cucumber
30g fresh wild mushroom
1/2 carrot
1/2 potato
10g ginger
2 slices of lemon
3 tbsp olive oil
1 tbsp sunflower oil
1/2 tbsp salt
2 tbsp oyster sauce
1/2 tsp white wine
1tbsp water

Method
1. Peel and cut the carrot and potato into large pieces. Peel and cut the ginger into large pieces. Cut the storks from the mushrooms. Marinate the scallops with wine in a bowl.

2. Put a wok on a maximum heat, add oil for a few seconds then add all the vegetables and mushrooms except the ginger. Stir for 8 minutes and add water if necessary. Add salt when done then bring everything onto a plate.

3. Put a non-stick frying pan on a maximum heat, add sunflower oil for a few seconds then add the scallops and sear each side, normally for 1-2 minutes, until

the surface of the scallop is light brown. Place the scallops on the plate, on top of the portion.

4. Place a slice of lemon on the side of the plate before serving.

100g Scallop nutrition information

Calories 88, Fat 0.76g, Sugar 0, Iron 2%

Yin and Yang score

Yang ++++ Yin ++

KING OF SPEECH

Ingredients:
1 whole sea bass, cleaned and gutted
80g firm tofu
5 black fungus
2 slices fresh lemon
10g ginger
10g spring onion
10g red chilli
3 tbsp olive oil
2 tbsp sesame oil
4 tbsp seasoned soy sauce for seafood
1 tsp salt
1 tsp red wine
1 tsp cider apple vinegar
4 tbsp water

Method
1. Soak and separate the black fungus leaves. Cut the firm tofu into square pieces. Cut the red chilli into rings. Peel and slice the ginger into pieces. Cut the spring onion into inch-long strips. Cut two slits in each side of the sea bass.

2. Mix the red wine, cider apple vinegar and seasoned soy sauce for sea food in a bowl.

3. Put kitchen foil on an oven tray, 2 1/2 times the size of the tray (be sure it can cover the whole seabass etc.) Place the seabass onto the kitchen foil then pour salt and oil over it. Place the ginger inside and outside

the sea bass. Pour the mixed sauce over the sea bass, add water around it, and add the black fungus and firm tofu on the side of the sea bass. Now close the foil, leaving an air gap inside the foil package. Bake in the oven at 150 degree for 30 minutes.

4. Bring the fish onto a plate.

5. Pour sesame oil onto the portion. Add sliced lemon to the side pf the plate before serving.

100g Sea Bream nutrition information

Calorie 96, Fat 2.9g, Sugar 0%, Iron 0%

Yin and Yang score

Yang +++++ Yin +++++

EVER POPULAR

Ingredient
250g fresh king prawn, shelled
10 dried black fungus
1/2 red chilli
10g ginger
10g garlic
20g spring onion
2 lemon slices
2 sunflower oil
1 tbsp sesame oil
1 tbsp premium light soy sauce
1 tsp cider apple vinegar
1/2 tsp salt
1/2 tsp white wine

Method
1. Peel and cut the ginger and garlic into small pieces.
   Chop the spring onion. Soak and chop the black
   fungus into small pieces. Chop the red chilli. Mix
   the king prawns with the wine and vinegar in
   a bowl.

2. Put a wok on a high heat, add oil for a few seconds
   then add the ginger and garlic for a few seconds
   before adding the black fungus and chilli together.
   Stir for 5 minutes then add the king prawns. Stir for
   2 minutes then add the salt and premium light soy
   sauce, stir for 3 minutes.

3. Bring everything to a plate, pour sesame oil over the

portion, and sprinkle with spring onion on the top before serving.

100g King prawn nutrition information
Calorie 105, Fat 2.2g, Sugar 2.2g, Iron 0

Yin and Yang score
Yang ++++ Yin +++

OLD FASHION

Ingredient
150g halibut
6 dried black fungus
1/2 cucumber
1/2 carrot
30g white radish
1/2 green bell pepper
10g ginger
10g coriander
2 tbsp olive oil
2 tbsp sunflower oil
1 tsp salt
2 tbsp seasoned soy sauce for sea food
1 tsp apple cider vinegar
1 tsp white wine
3 tbsp water

Method
1. Slice the halibut into large pieces. Cut the cucumber and green bell pepper into medium pieces. Peel and cut the carrot and white radish into medium pieces. Soak and cut the dry black fungus into medium pieces. Peel and slice the ginger. Chop up the coriander.

2. Mix the white wine, vinegar, seasoned soy sauce and sesame oil together in a bowl to create a sauce.

3. Put a wok on a high heat, add sunflower oil for a few seconds then add all the vegetables except the

a coriander, and stir for 5 minutes. Add salt about 2 minutes before it is ready. Add water if necessary to prevent drying or burning. Then bring everything onto a plate

4. Put a non-stick frying pan onto a maximum heat, add the olive oil for a few seconds, then add the halibut and cook on both sides till light brown. Bring everything on the top of the portion.

5. Put a wok on a maximum heat again, add the mixed sauce with 3 tbsp water for a few seconds until boiling then pour it on the portion.

6. Sprinkle coriander over the portion before serving.

100g Halibut nutrition information

Calorie 110, Fat 2.29g, Sugar 0, Iron 55%

Yin and Yang score

Yang +++++ Yin +++

All these recipes can be eaten as an evening meal

Meat recipes

- Portion: 1-2 people
- Preparation time: 10-25 minutes
- During cooking, add a little water if necessary to prevent drying out or burning.

ANGEL SPARKLING FLOWER

Ingredient

100g chicken mince
120g broccoli or cauliflower florets
10g spring onion
10g ginger
20g red bell pepper
1 tsp oyster sauce
2 tbsp light soy sauce
1 tsp white wine
2 tbsp olive oil
1 tbsp sesame oil
1 tsp salt
water

Method

1. Cut the broccoli or cauliflower florets in half. Dice the spring onion. Cut the red bell pepper into small pieces. Peel and cut the ginger into small pieces. Mix the chicken mince and wine together.

2. Add the broccoli or cauliflower florets to a pan of

boiling water for 5 minutes, rinse in a sieve under the tap water then place on a plate.

3. Put a wok on a maximum heat, add olive oil for a few seconds then add the ginger and spring onion for a few seconds, before adding the red bell pepper and chicken mince together. Stir for 8 minutes then add the salt, light soy sauce and oyster sauce together, and stir for a further 3 minutes. Add water if necessary to prevent drying or burning.

4. Bring everything onto the plate on top of the broccoli cauliflower florets.

5. Pour sesame oil onto the portion before serving.

100g Chicken mince nutrition information

Calories 134, Fat 6g, Sugar 1g, Iron 0%

Yin and Yang Score

Yang ++++ Yin +++

MIDDLE AUTUMN

Ingredients
100 turkey breast, without skin
160g red bell pepper
100g white radish
3 dried black mushroom
10g spring onion
10g ginger
2 tbsp olive oil
2 tbsp sunflower oil
1 tsp salt
1 tsp white wine
1 tbsp premium light soy sauce
1 tsp cider apple vinegar
3 tbsp water

Method

1. Cut the red bell pepper, peeled white radish, spring onion and peeled ginger into strips. Soak the dried black mushroom and cut into strips. Cut the turkey breast into pieces and mix with wine and vinegar in a bowel.

2. Put a wok on a maximum heat, add sunflower oil for a few seconds then add all the vegetables and the black mushroom, except for the spring onion. Stir for 10 minutes, then bring to a plate.

3. Put a wok on a maximum heat again, add olive oil for a few seconds then add the ginger and spring onion for a few seconds, before adding the turkey breast

with wine and vinegar. Stir for 5 minutes then bring the cooked vegetables back to the wok and add the premium light soy sauce and salt. Stir for 5 minutes. Add water if necessary to prevent drying or burning.

4. Bring everything onto a plate and serve.

100g Turkey breast nutrition information
Calories 104, Fat 1.66g, Sugar 3.51g, Iron 8%

Yin and Yang Score
Yang ++++ Yin +++

AMAZING CONCERT

Ingredient
100g skinless chicken breast
8 dried black fungus
160g cucumber
10g ginger
10g spring onion
3 tbsp olive oil
2 tbsp sunflower oil
1/2 tsp salt
2 tbsp premium light soy sauce
1 tsp white wine
1 tsp vinegar
3 tbsp water

Method

1. Slice the chicken breast into large angled pieces then mix with the wine and vinegar in a bowl. Cut the cucumber and peeled ginger into large pieces. Soak and cut the dry black fungus into large pieces. Cut the spring onion into strips.

2. Put a wok on a maximum heat, add olive oil for a few seconds then add the ginger and spring onion for a few seconds before adding the chicken breast. Stir for 5 minutes then add the black fungus and cucumber. Stir for 5 minutes then add the salt and premium light soy sauce. Stir for a further 5 minutes. Add water if necessary to prevent drying or burning.

3. It is ready to serve.

100g Chicken breast nutrition information
Calories 165, Fat 3.6g, Sugar 0, Iron 5%

Yin and Yang Score
Yang +++++ Yin +++

ORIGINAL ELEMENT

Ingredients
100g pork mince
30g long kou bean noodles
4 pak choi
10 goji Berries
10g ginger
10g spring onion
2tbsp olive oil
2tbsp sunflower oil
1tbsp oyster sauce
1tbsp premium light soy sauce
1tsp salt
1tsp wine (red or white)
1tsp cider apple vinegar
water

Method
1. Cut the pak choi down the middle. Soak the goji berries. Chop the spring onion into small pieces. Peel and dice the ginger into small pieces. Soak and rinse the long kou bean noodles. Marinate the minced pork with the white wine and vinegar in a bowl.

2. Put a wok on a maximum heat, add sunflower oil for few seconds then add 1/2 tsp salt and the pak choi. Stir for 5 minutes then bring everything onto a plate.

3. Put a non-stick pan on a maximum heat, add olive oil for a few seconds then add the ginger and spring onion for few seconds. Add the minced pork and stir for 5 minutes, then add the long kou bean noodles

and stir for a further 8 minutes. Add 1/2 tsp salt, premium light soy sauce and oyster sauce together, and stir for 2 minutes. In the meantime, add water if necessary to prevent drying or burning. Bring everything onto the plate on top of the cooked pak choi.

4. Sprinkle the goji berries on top to serve.

100g Pork mince nutrition information

Calories 161, Fat 7g, Sugar 0g, Iron 0.9g

Yin and Yang score

Yang +++++ Yin +++

WONDERFUL WORLD

Ingredient
100g beef mince
100g echalion shallot mushrooms
100g courgettes
100 carrot
10g ginger
10g spring onion
1tsp salt
3 tbsp olive oil
1tbsp premium light soy sauce
1tsp wine (red or white)
1tsp cider apple vinegar
1 tbsp water

Method
1. Cut the storks off the echalion shallot mushrooms. Angle slice the courgettes. Peel and slice the carrots and ginger. Cut the spring onion into strips. Mix the minced beef with the wine and vinegar in a bowl.

2. Put a wok on a maximum heat, add olive oil for a few seconds then add the ginger and spring onion for a few seconds before adding the minced beef. Stir for 5 minutes. Put the beef into a bowl but keep the oil in the wok. Then add the courgettes and carrot back to the wok and stir for 8 minutes before adding the echalion shallot mushrooms, salt and premium light soy sauce together. Continue to stir for 2 minutes then add the cooked minced beef, and stir for 2 more

minutes. Add water if necessary to prevent drying or burning.

3. Bring all things to the plate and serve.

100g Beef mince nutrition information
Calories 332, Fat 30g, Sugar 0g, Iron 8%

Yin and Yang score
Yang +++++ Yin ++++

COUNTRY STYLISH

Ingredient

100g pork chops

100g Chinese leaf

100g chestnut mushrooms

80g green bell pepper

1/2 red chilli

10g ginger

5g spring onions

3 tbsp olives oil

2 tbsp sunflower oil

1 tsp salt

1 tbsp light soy sauce

1 tbsp oyster sauce

1 tsp wine (red or white)

1 tsp cider apple vinegar

1 tbsp water

Method

1. Peel and slice the ginger into large pieces. Cut the Chinese leaf into large pieces. Cut the chestnut mushrooms, green bell pepper and red chilli together into large pieces. Cut the spring onion into strips. Slice the pork chops into large angled pieces then mix with wine and cider apple vinegar in a bowl.

2. Put a wok on a maximum heat, add sunflower oil for a few seconds then add all the vegetables except for the spring onion and ginger. Stir for 5 minutes then bring everything into a bowl.

3. Put a wok on a maximum heat, add olive oil for a few seconds then add the ginger and spring onion for a few seconds before adding the pork chops. Stir for 8 minutes then add the light soy sauce and stir for 2 minutes. Bring all the cooked vegetables back to the wok, add the salt and oyster sauce then stir for a further 5 minutes. In the meantime, add water if necessary to prevent drying or burning.

4. It is ready to serve.

100g Pork chops nutrition information

Calories 231, Fat 14g, Sugar 0g, Iron 4%

Yin and Yang score

Yang +++++ Yin ++++

TIMELESS FASHION

Ingredients
100g beef steak
100g firm tofu
100g celery
5 dried black mushroom
1/2 red chilli
10g ginger
10g spring onion
1/2 tsp salt
3 tbsp olive oil
2 tbsp sunflower oil
2 tbsp light soy sauce
1 tbsp oyster sauce
1 tsp wine (red or white)
1 tbsp cider apple vinegar
3 tbsp water

Method
1. Cut the celery, tofu, peeled ginger and spring onion into strips. Soak and cut the dried black mushroom into pieces. Take out the seeds from the red chilli and cut them into strips. Slice the beef into strips and mix with wine and vinegar in a bowl.

2. Put a wok on a maximum heat, add sunflower oil for a few seconds then add the celery, tofu, black mushroom and red chilli together. Stir for 8 minutes, adding water as necessary to prevent the vegetables drying or burning, then bring everything to a bowl.

3. Put a wok on a maximum heat, add olive oil for a few seconds then add the ginger and spring onion for a few seconds before adding the beef. Stir for 5 minutes. Turn the heat down to medium, bring all the cooked vegetables back to the wok and add the oyster sauce, light soy sauce and salt. Stir for 8 minutes.

4. It is ready to serve.

100g Beef steak nutrition information
Calories 271, Fat 19g, Sugar 0g, Iron 13%

Yin and Yang score
Yang +++++ Yin ++++

All these recipes can be served as an evening meal

EVENING WEIGHT LOSS RECIPES

SOUP

- Portion: 2-3 people
- Preparation time: 10-15 minutes

EGG AND BABY PAK CHOI SOUP

Ingredient

1 egg
1 baby pak choi
10g ginger
1 tbsp sunflower oil
1/2 tsp salt
500ml boiling water

Method

1. Chop the baby pak choi. Whisk the egg in a bowl. Peel and slice the ginger.

2. Put a pan of boiling water on a medium heat then add the baby pak choi, ginger and oil and simmer for 4 minutes. Then add the whisked egg and salt for a few seconds and stir.

3. It is ready to serve.

100g Egg nutrition information

Calories 155, Fat 15g, Sugar 1.1g, Iron 6%

Yin and Yang score

Yang ++++ Yin +++

TOFU AND CORIANDER SOUP

Ingredients
80g silk tofu
5g coriander
10g ginger
1/2 tsp salt
1 tbsp sunflower oil
500 ml boiling water

Method
1. Slice the tofu. Peel and slice the ginger. Chop the coriander into pieces.

2. Put a pan of boiling water on a medium heat then add the tofu, ginger and sunflower oil. Simmer for 5 minutes then add the coriander and salt for a few seconds.

3. It is ready to serve.

100g Silk tofu nutrition information
Calories 55, Fat 2.7g, Sugar 1.31g, Iron 5%

Yin and Yang score
Yang ++++ Yin ++++

CHICKEN AND CHINESE CABBAGE SOUP

Ingredients

30g chicken breast without skin

30g Chinese cabbage

10g spring onion

10g ginger

1/2 salt

1tbsp sunflower oil

1tbsp light soy sauce

1tsp wine

500ml boiled water

Method

1. Chop the chicken breast then mix with the wine in a bowl. Chop the Chinese cabbage and spring onion. Peel and dice the ginger.

2. Put a pan of boiling water on a medium heat then add the chicken, Chinese cabbage, ginger and oil. Simmer for 8 minutes then add the salt, soy sauce and spring onion together, and simmer for a few seconds.

3. It is ready to serve.

100g Sunflower oil nutrition information

Calories 884, Fat 100g, Sugar 0%, Iron 0 %

Yin and Yang score

Yang ++++ Yin +

BEEF AND RADISH SOUP

Ingredients
30g beef fillet
50g white radish
10g celery leaf
10g ginger
1/2 tsp salt
1tbsp sunflower oil
1tsp light soy sauce
1tsp wine
500ml boiled water

Method
1. Slice the beef and marinate with the red wine in a bowl. Peel and slice the white radish. Peel and chop the ginger. Chop the celery leaves.

2. Put a pan of boiling water on a medium heat then add the radish, celery, ginger and oil, and simmer for 8 minutes. Then add the beef and simmer for a further 5 minutes, before adding the light soy sauce and salt for a few seconds.

3. It is ready to serve.

100g White radish nutrition information
Calories 18, Fat 0.1g, Sugar 2.5g , Iron 2%

Yin and Yang score
Yang ++++ Yin +++++

PRAWN AND MUSHROOM SOUP

Ingredients
30g peeled prawns
60g enoki mushroom
1/3 cucumber
10g spring onion
10g ginger
1/2 tsp salt
1 tsp sunflower oil
1 tsp light soy sauce
2 cups (500ml) water

Method
1. Chop the peeled prawns. Chop the mushroom, spring onion and cucumber. Peel and chop the ginger.

2. Put a pan of boiling water on a medium heat then add the cucumber, enoki mushroom, ginger and oil. Simmer for 10 minutes then add the prawns and simmer for 3 minutes. Then add the salt and spring onion for a few seconds.

3. It is ready to serve.

100g Enoki mushroom nutrition information
Calories 45, Fat 0.4g, Sugar 0.22g, Iron 6%

Yin and Yang score
Yang ++++ Yin +++++

COD FILLET AND PLUM TOMATOES

Ingredients
30g cod fillet
30g plum tomatoes
10g chives
10g ginger
1/2 tsp salt
1tbsp sunflower oil
1tsp light soy sauce
1tsp wine (red or white)
2 cups (500ml) water

Method
1. Chop the cod fillet and mix with the wine in a bowl. Chop the plum tomatoes and chives. Peel and chop the ginger.

2. Put a pan of boiling water on a medium heat then add the plum tomatoes, ginger and oil. Simmer for 10 minutes then add the cod fillet pieces and simmer for 2 minutes. Then add the light soy sauce and salt for a few seconds.

3. Sprinkle chives on the top before serving.

100g Cod fillet nutrition information

Calories 82, Fat 0.7g, Sugar 0g, Iron 2%

Yin and Yang score

Yang ++++ Yin +++

SEAWEED AND CUCUMBER SOUP

Ingredients
3g dried seaweed
40g cucumber
15g carrot
3g chives
1/2 tsp salt
1 tsp sunflower oil
2 cups (500ml) water

Method
1. Peel and angle slice the carrot. Angle slice the cucumber. Cut the chives into small pieces.

2. Put a pan of boiling water on a medium heat then add the cucumber, carrot and sunflower oil. Simmer for 8 minutes then add the chives, dried seaweed and salt. Stir using chopsticks for a few seconds, to separate the seaweed leaves into the soup.

3. It is ready to serve.

100g Seaweed nutrition information
Calories 43, Fat 0.6g, Sugar 0.6g, Iron 16%

Yin and Yang score
Yang ++++ Yin+++++

These soups can be served for lunch. You can always add different vegetables, egg or meat. Soup is particularly good if you are recovering from sickness or surgery

Vegetarian Recipes

- Portion: 1-2 people
- Preparation time: 10-25 minutes
- During cooking, add a little water if necessary to prevent drying out or burning.

PEACOCK

Ingredients

160g sweet stemmed cauliflower
10 dried black mushrooms
5g goji berries
15g garlic
10g ginger
1tsp salt
2tbsp olive oil
1tsp sesame oil
1 tbsp oyster soy sauce
1/2 tsp cider apple vinegar
3 tbsp water

Method

1. Peel and dice the garlic and ginger. Soak and chop the dried black mushrooms. Chop the sweet stemmed cauliflower. Soak the goji berries for 10 minutes.

2. Put a pan of boiling water on a maximum heat

then add the sweet stemmed cauliflower, cook for 5 minutes then sieve under tap water before putting onto a plate.

3. Put a wok on a maximum heat, add oil for a few seconds then add the ginger for a few seconds. Then add the mushrooms and stir for 5 minutes. Turn the heat down to medium then add the oyster soy sauce, vinegar, salt and water, and slowly cook for 10 minutes. Then turn the heat back to maximum for a few seconds, making sure the sauce is thick and creamy.

4. Bring everything to the plate of cauliflower. Pour the sesame oil on top before serving.

100g Sweet stemmed cauliflower nutrition information
Calories 25, Fat 0.1g, Sugar 2.4g, Iron 2%

Yin and Yang Score
Yang + Yin ++++

SEASON GREETING

Ingredients

200g asparagus

10 scallops

10g walnuts

10g ginger

2 slices of lemon

3 tbsp sunflower oil

1/2 tbsp olive oil

1/2 tsp salt

3 tbsp premium light soy sauce

250ml boiling water

Method

1. Cut the asparagus into inch-long pieces. Rinse the scallops. Crush the walnuts. Peel and dice the ginger.

2. Put a pan of boiling water on a maximum heat, then add the asparagus and cook for 5 minutes. Sieve with tap water and put them on a plate.

3. Put a non-stick frying pan on a maximum heat, add 1 tbsp sunflower oil, making sure the oil has spread out. Add the ginger for a few seconds then turn the heat down to medium, add the scallops and cook on each side for 1-2 minutes until golden brown. Place the scallops on the top of the asparagus on the plate. Now add the rest of the sunflower oil, salt, premium light soy sauce and 1tbsp water in the same pan for a couple minutes, making sure the sauce is thick and creamy.

4. Pour the sauce on top of the asparagus and sprinkle with the crushed walnuts before serving.

5. Add a squeeze of lemon if desired.

100g Asparagus nutrition information
Calories 20, Fat 0.1, Sugar 1.9, Iron 11%

Yin and Yang score
Yang +++ Yin +++++

FOUR SEASON

Ingredients
6 (150g) baby pak choi
60g fresh mixed wild mushrooms
20g garlic
10g ginger
2 tbsp olive oil
1 tbsp sesame oil
1/2 tsp salt
2 tbsp premium light soy sauce
1 tbsp water

Method
1. Cut the baby pak choi into pieces. Cut off the mushroom storks. Crush the garlic. Peel and slice the ginger.

2. Put a wok on a maximum heat then add the olive oil and ginger for a few seconds before adding the baby pak choi and mushrooms. Stir for 5 minutes then add the salt and premium light soy sauce for a couple of minutes. Add water if necessary to prevent drying or burning. Bring everything onto a plate.

3. Put the same wok on a maximum heat again then add the sesame oil and garlic for a few seconds. Then pour this sauce on top of the vegetables and mushrooms.

4. It is ready to serve.

100g Garlic nutrition information

Calories 149, Fat 1g, Sugar 1g, Iron 9%

Yin and Yang score

Yang +++ Yin +

EVER FASHION

Ingredients
2 eggs
180g tomatoes
10 spring onion
3 tbsp sunflower oil
1/2 tsp salt
1/2 tsp wine (red or white)
2 cups (500ml) water

Method
1. Cut the spring onion into small pieces, then break the eggs into a bowl and whisk.

2. Add the tomatoes to a pan of boiling water for 2 minutes then rinse under tap water, peel the skin off and cut into slices, then bring them to a plate.

3. Put a wok on a medium heat, add sunflower oil for a few seconds then pour the eggs into the wok, stirring softly for a couple of minutes. Then bring the cooked eggs on top of the tomatoes.

4. Sprinkle spring onion on top of the eggs before serving.

100g Tomatoes nutrition information
Calories 18, Fat 0.2g, Sugar 2.6g, Iron 1%

Yin and Yang score
Yang +++ Yin +++++

EVER LOVE

Ingredients
180g long green sweet pepper
50g shiitake mushrooms
15g garlic
2tbsp sunflower oil
1tbsp sesame oil
1/2tsp salt
1tbsp light soy sauce
2tbsp oyster sauce

Method
1. Slice the peppers and shiitake mushrooms. Peel and crush the garlic.

2. Put a wok on a maximum heat, add sunflower oil for a few seconds then add the peppers and shiitake mushrooms. Stir for 8 minutes then add the salt and light soy sauce. Continue to stir for a couple minutes then bring everything onto to a plate. Now, using same the wok, add the sesame oil and garlic for a few seconds then pour them over the portion.

3. It is ready to serve.

100g Long green sweet pepper
Calories 26, Fat 0.3g, Sugar 4.2g, Iron 2%

Yin and Yang score
Yang ++ Yin ++++

ORCHESTRA

Ingredients
1 peeled medium size beetroot
50g fresh garden peas
30 baby sweet corn
6 chestnut mushrooms
30g peeled carrots
50g peeled white radish
100g firm tofu
10 black olives
3 tbsp olive oil
1 tsp salt
1 tbsp light soy sauce
3 tbsp water

Method
1. Chop and dice the beetroot, baby corn and chestnut mushrooms. Peel and chop the carrot and white radish. Chop the tofu.

2. Put a wok on a maximum heat, add oil for a few seconds then add the baby corn, chestnut mushrooms, carrot, white radish and fresh garden peas. Stir for 10 minutes then add the tofu and stir for 3 minutes before adding the salt and light soy sauce. Stir for 5 minutes then add the beetroot for a couple of minutes. Add water if necessary to prevent drying or burning.

3. It is ready to serve.

100g Beetroot nutrition information
Calories 43, Fat 0.2g, Sugar 7.g, Iron 4%

Yin and Yang score
Yang +++ Yin +++++

SUMMER SEASON
(with or without chicken)

Ingredients:
200g cucumber
150g chicken breast
30g dried black fungus
3g coriander
10g ginger
3 tbsp olive oil
1/2 tsp salt
1/2 tsp white wine
1/2 tsp apple cider vinegar

Method:
1. Slice the cucumber into large pieces. Soak the dried black fungus and rinse. Chop the coriander into strips. Peel and chop the ginger. Slice the chicken breast and mix with the wine and vinegar in a bowl.

2. Put a wok on a maximum heat, add oil for a few seconds then add the ginger for a few seconds before adding the chicken pieces. Stir for 5 minutes then bring the chicken to a plate. Keep the oil in the wok and add the cucumber and black fungus, stirring for 8 minutes. Bring the cooked chicken back to the wok and add salt then stir for a couple of minutes.

3. Sprinkle coriander onto the portion before serving.

100g Cucumber nutrition information
Calories 16, Sugar 1.7g, Iron 1%, Vitamin C 4%

Yin and Yang Score
Yang ++ Yin +++++

These recipes can also be served for lunch

7 DAY RECIPE WEIGHT LOSS DIET PLAN

Here is a simple 7 day plan that you can follow to help you start to lose weight. Remember:

- Each day, you need to follow the daily rotation of A.B.C.D
- Before a meal, you should drink tea (cold, hot, or Chinese tea)
- After a meal, you should have a piece of fruit
- For lunch or evening, you should have a portion of steamed rice to accompany your meal

DAY 1

Breakfast
- Goji Berries Rice Porridge (see page 154 for recipe)
- 2 Hard-boiled medium size eggs

Lunch
- Tofu and Chinese Cabbage Soup (see page 175 for recipe)
- Angel Sparkling Flower (see page 207 for recipe)

Evening
- Egg and Baby Pak Choi Soup (see page 221 for recipe)
- Aubergines (see page 185 for recipe)

DAY 2

Breakfast

- Sliced Eggs with Cucumber (see page 162 for recipe)
- Mixed Dry Nuts (150ml) (see page 171 for recipe)

Lunch

- Tofu and Dry Seaweed Soup (see page 177 for recipe)
- Village Fish (see page 195 for recipe)

Evening

- Tofu and Coriander Soup (see page 222 for recipe)
- Season Greeting (see page 230 for recipe)

DAY 3

Breakfast

- Fried Rice and Tofu (see page 166 for recipe)
- Vegetable Drink (150ml) (see page 174 for recipe)

Lunch

- White Radish and Exotic Mushroom Soup (see page 178 for recipe)
- Silk Tofu Bao (see page 183 for recipe)

Evening

- Prawn and Mushroom Soup (see page 225 for recipe)
- Four Season (see page 232 for recipe)

DAY 4

Breakfast

- Sweetcorn Rice Porridge (see page 156 for recipe)
- Poached Eggs with Tomato (see page 163 for recipe)

Lunch

- Spinach Soup (see page 179 for recipe)
- Middle Autumn (see page 209 for recipe)

Evening

- Chicken and Chinese Cabbage Soup (see page 223 for recipe)
- Ever Fashion (see page 234 for recipe)

DAY 5

Breakfast

- Shiitake Mushroom Rice Porridge (see page 158 for recipe)
- Stir-Steam Eggs (see page 164 for recipe)

Lunch

- Pork Soup (see page 180 for recipe)
- Romantic Cod (see page 197 for recipe)

Evening

- Beef and Radish Soup (see page 224 for recipe)
- Ever Love (see page 235 for recipe)

DAY 6

Breakfast

- Fried Rice and Shrimps (see page 168 for recipe)
- Mixed Dry Nuts (see page 171 for recipe)

Lunch

- Baby Corn Soup (see page 181 for recipe)
- Disney Beauty (see page 198 for recipe)

Evening

- Cod Fillet and Plum Tomatoes (see page 226 for recipe)
- Orchestra (see page 236 for recipe)

DAY 7

Breakfast

- Chicken Rice Porridge (see page 160 for recipe)
- Stir-Steam Eggs (see page 164 for recipe)

Lunch

- Kale and Eryngii Mushroom Soup (see page 182 for recipe)
- Old Beauty (see page 199 for recipe)

Evening

- Seaweed and Cucumber Soup (see page 227 for recipe)
- Middle Autumn (see page 209 for recipe)

CHAPTER 8

Popular Chinese Exercises and Meditation

M any Chinese people know that diet is vital for a healthy and slim lifestyle, but the importance of incorporating physical exercise into a daily routine should never be neglected. This thinking is apparent throughout Chinese philosophy.

Confucius (a Chinese social philosopher) was fond of swimming, mountain climbing and archery. Laozi, the founder of Taoism, favoured Qigong, which is the foundation of Chinese martial arts. Kangxi, the longest ruling Emperor in Chinese history, loved horse riding and shooting.

Traditional Chinese exercises have been studied for at least 2000 years. In contrast to the modern Western approach, traditional Chinese self-practice exercises do not focus on pushing the body to its physical limits. Instead, the emphasis is on consistency and perseverance.

Moderate and gentle flowing activities are considered the best way to move Qi and blood around the body to achieve health, harmony and an overall sense of wellbeing. The exercises tend to focus on loosening, stretching and relaxing the body and involve a controlled, regulated breathing pattern.

Taoists believe that life is not measured in years, but rather breaths and heartbeats. Therefore, exercise is not about getting the heart racing; it is about inviting the Qi to flow, opening the body by focussing on joints and muscles associated with the spinal column. The spine is the largest micro-system in the body, so loosening and stretching these vertebrae and softening the spinal muscles restores optimum nerve and energy impulses to the vital organs.

Traditional Chinese exercises are still popular today. Take a morning walk through almost any park in China and you'll see people of different ages (even those in their 90s) practising a daily workout routine of stretching, strengthening, breathing and self-massage.

Try doing some of these traditional exercises instead of going to the gym.

The Five Animal Play

The five animal play, also known as 'remedy dancing', is a classic set of Qigong exercises inspired by the movement of five animals: tiger, deer, bear, monkey and crane. By mimicking the animals' behaviour, practitioners cultivate energy to use in daily life and gain strength, flexibility, balance and coordination.

TIGER MOVEMENT

Take a deep breath and clench fists. Look down and swoop fists to the right and left sides repeatedly. Stretch the body and raise arms slowly as if lifting an extremely heavy object. While doing this, gulp down breath soundly.

DEER MOVEMENT

Raise your head and shake it to the left and right sides repeatedly. Steer your body in alternate directions while looking down, as if chasing your tail. Hold your breath, clench fists, stretch the body as far as possible and jump up on tiptoes.

BEAR MOVEMENT

Sway from the waist while striding towards the left side and then right side to mimic a bear walking. Stand up straight and make the joints crack.

MONKEY MOVEMENT

Hold your breath and position yourself like a monkey climbing a tree. Stretch out one hand as if grasping a fruit and have one leg raised; make the other leg twist with the body while gulping down the breath until you start to sweat.

CRANE MOVEMENT

Take another deep breath. Bow the body and raise your head like a bird preparing to take a flight. Lift arms just above the head and touch fingertips together, gently stroking from the forehead to nose. Then lightly tap the crown of the head with your fingers.

There are several variations and movements in the five animal play. Many can be found on the *PetarSmilijana Qigong Channel:* (www.youtube.com/watch?v=-x8QrpDPGE). For the best results, we recommend learning from a professional practitioner.

The Wand Exercises

This is another ancient Chinese practice related to the martial arts. The wand is a 48-50 inches long dowel (wooden pole) 1 inch in diameter, often made of wood or bamboo. It's used as a fulcrum for balance, form and posture, putting the practitioner in the centre. There are hundreds of wand exercises, but focus on 17 gentle bending, twisting and lunging routines specially designed to get blood circulating more efficiently throughout the body.

These 17 exercises use every major muscle in the body and take no more than 20 minutes to complete. They provide a more efficient method of staying fit and healthy by increasing and balancing the chi (Qi) energy.

You can learn the 17 wand exercises from the Grand Master Brunce L Johnson's book 'Chinese Wand Exercise'.

Michael Davies also published a series of videos on his blog: https://michaeldaviesuk.wordpress.com/the-17-exercises/

There are many more exercises we can discuss, but in general, cycling, dancing, hiking and rope skipping are recommended as good forms of daily exercises.

To conclude, the secret to Chinese slimming exercises is not to push your body to its limit or train your muscles to the extreme. Instead, try to incorporate gentle, flowing exercises into your daily life to strengthen and tone in the long run.

Chinese Meditation

Hui, a disciple of Confucius, once said: 'I venture to ask what "fasting of the mind" is.'

Confucius replied: 'Maintaining the unity of your will. Listen not with your ears but with your mind. Listen not with your mind but with your primal breath. The ears are limited to listening, the mind is limited to tallying. The primal breath, however, awaits things emptily. It is only through the Way that one can gather emptiness, and emptiness is the fasting of the mind.'

Chinese Meditation was developed around 500-600 BCE and has its roots in Chinese Buddhism, 'Chan' teaching and Chinese philosophical theories such as Taoism. The four key focuses are concentration, mindfulness, contemplation, and visualization.

Here are a few important terms:

'Ding' – means 'decide, settle, stabilize, definite, firm, solid.'

'Guan' – means 'look carefully watch, observe, view, scrutinize.'

'Cun' – means 'exist, be present, live, survive, remain.'

'Zuowang' – means 'sitting and forgetting.'

'Shouyi' – means 'guarding the one; maintaining oneness.'

'Yuanyou' – means 'far-off journey; ecstatic excursion.'

There are three stages in practising Chinese meditation. The first stage of practice is learning to sit in a settle way with clarity and simplicity in the moment to achieve a 'concentrated mind'.

The second stage is to open your field of awareness, connecting your body with the external environment. The external environment should pose no opposition or burden. It's what it is, sitting with you. Through this, you can achieve a 'unified mind'.

The third stage is realization of quiescence and wakefulness, stillness and awareness. It's the stage of enlightenment –'no self, no mind' – returning to the original natural peaceful state of mind.

Zuochan

Zuochan, also called 'Zazen' (in Japan) or 'seated Zen' is the most important form of Chinese meditation.

Zuochan is generally practised seated on the floor on a mat and cushion with crossed legs. Traditionally it was done in the lotus or half lotus position.

The most important thing is to keep the back completely straight, from the pelvis to the neck. The mouth is kept close and eyes remain lowered, with your gaze resting on the ground about two or three feet in front of you.

Focus all your attention on the movement of breath going in and out through the nose. To help, silently count down the number of breaths, from 10 to 1. Then start the process again. If you get distracted and lose count, gently bring back the attention to 10 and resume from there.

Practitioners remain as much as possible in the present moment, aware of and observing what passes through their minds and around them, without dwelling on anything in particular.

The first stage of a deeply concentrated mind is most easy to achieve. We recommend combining Zuochan exercises with the physical exercises in the previous chapter for the best results.

Chinese meditation does not focus on any specific practice or position; it's about creating harmony within yourself and connecting with your environment to achieve knowledge through reflection and contemplation. The goal of meditation is to mature as a person, to relax and become fully aware of yourself and the world around you. It's a road that leads to self-knowledge and awareness.

CHAPTER 9

Stay Slim Forever

As a practitioner of Traditional Chinese Medicine for over 30 years, I've treated a broad range of health issues. But for the past 15 years, I have specialised in weight loss and management. This book arose from my experience as a practitioner, both in the UK and China, and the growing number of clients I meet who have experienced weight problems or excessive weight caused by other health issues.

I have come to understand the underlying reasons for these weight and health problems and why they are so common in the West, and this book is based on the insights, knowledge and experience I have gained in this field.

The purpose of my book is to enlighten people on a way of eating and living that enables them to:

- Maintain a healthy weight or keep slim
- Lose weight if they need to
- Live a healthy and balanced life

My approach and the focus of my book is based on the Traditional Chinese Medicine philosophy of Yin and Yang balance and how you can apply it to your diet and lifestyle:

- Be introduced to the Chinese way of living where you'll learn to understand the philosophy of Yin and Yang balance and discover the benefits of following the Chinese approach in terms of diet and lifestyle
- Uncover the secrets behind why the Chinese nation are able to stay so slim and healthy even in their old age and find out why Westerners are so prone to diet and lifestyle-related health problems
- Master your daily cycle to get the most from working, eating, sleeping, exercising and socialising
- Find more ways you can use Yin and Yang balance to improve other areas of your life

The book explores how all the things in your life can influence and affect each other, how they can be disturbed and how Yin and Yang can become unbalanced, and what you can do to regain your balance.

The Chinese see food as medicine, it is a central aspect

for achieving balance and food is also at the core of losing weight and living a healthy lifestyle. Knowledge of how different foods interact and can affect your body's energy is also crucial, and an important step towards achieving a truly balanced diet.

It is often the case that people fail to reach their weight loss goal or even complete their weight loss journey. The book provides you with answers to why this happens, common mistakes made when losing weight and how you can make sure to avoid them to reach your goal.

The book also covers nutrition as well as the concepts that govern the Chinese approach to healthy eating and why it is so different to the West. Learn to identify foods that:

- Are easy to digest
- Eliminate toxins from the body
- Help your body maintain its natural energy
- Help you maintain a healthy weight

Finally the book also offers plenty of recipes for you to choose from. Whether your making a snack, breakfast, lunch or dinner they are all easy to follow, with detailed ingredients and a step by step guide to help you.

So join this Chinese life journcy, and find how to lead a healthier, happier life where you won't just lose weight but learn how to maintain it.

.

Acknowledgements

Since arriving in London 15 years ago it has been my dream to publicize the benefits of living according to the principles of Traditional Chinese Medicine. As a clinician, I have treated many patients suffering from a variety of health problems resulting from their diet and lifestyle. These problems can be avoided by living according to the principles of Yin and Yang balance as it relates to lifestyle, diet, exercise, work life balance, sleep and social activities.

Thankful clients whom I have been able to help have often said to me, 'You should write a book on the Chinese philosophy of life and Chinese life more generally. It is something we would like to know more about.'

I have been very busy running my TCM Practice and improving my English. It is only now that I have been able to write this book, *The Yin Yang Guide to Weight Loss*.

In doing this I have been helped by my editor, clients and colleagues, friends and family. Without them, my dream would not have come true.

I wish to thank the distinguished author and Sociologist, Lord Giddens (Anthony Giddens). He was the first person to tell me I could be a writer. He gave me a Christmas gift of a 4th edition of his book *Sociology*, in 2006 and reading this book gave me the self-belief and strength to build a successful business in England.

My thanks to Tony Parsons. He made me gifts of his best-selling novels, *Man and Boy*, *One for my Baby*, and *Man and Wife* in 2007. Reading these really helped me improve my English. Tony inspired me with his spirit and his success. There is a Chinese saying, 'Right person you meet, right path that will become clear to you'. I understood from him that it was not necessary to speak excellent academic English to write my book – the key thing was to be able to communicate well.

Kevin Shields is a musician with the band My Bloody Valentine, He encouraged me to take English lessons. I now thank him for that very good advice. Doing those lessons helped me develop my communication skills, enabled me to undertake further studies and was another step towards the writing of this book.

I am very grateful to John Blake, the British journalist. He introduced me to my Editor, Ciara Lloyd. Her advice was very helpful. She and Sarah Marshall's assistance is helping me to realize my dream.

My good friend, Maureen Ursich, has helped me personally and with my English. She has been the first to read this book and has helped me bring more clarity to my message.

I have been very fortunate in having assistance from a great team of students from Westminster University, the London School of Economics and the Traditional Chinese Medicine Department of Jilin University, namely: Junyi Wang, Tianci Cai and Zezhou Yan. They have helped me with research and been hugely supportive whilst I focus on completing this book.

My appreciation and thanks to Miss Kofoworola Ogungbayi, Miss Samar Abdel Rahman, Miss Vivan Xu, and Miss Wen Zhu who helped my English during Christmas time.

I also wish to thank my clients who have given me so much support and placed their trust in Traditional Chinese Medicine including, Chris Furr (Artist), Richard Park (Media Personality), Jocelyn Brown (Singer-Songwriter), Cherry Lena Chin, Tracy Miller, Susan Yuang and all those who have advised and supported me.

It has been a privilege to study and work with many distinguished experts and professors in Traditional Chinese Medicine, including Yumei Zhao, Allan Tran, Xiangping Zhang, Naming Chen, Yanhua Jing, and Jiangling Lu. I have learned from their depth of knowledge and experience and been impressed by their care of and commitment to their clients. Words do not express how much I appreciate the support they have given me.

My daughter Amy, my sister-in-law Christine, and my partner Peter have listened to my ideas and ambitions for this book and have read my early drafts. Their love and support has sustained me – particularly at those times when I have wondered if there was a Western audience for a book of this kind. I am grateful to Amy and Peter for taking the photographs which appear in this book.

I would like to remember my parents and my family in China. My parents who have now passed, they were my greatest supporters and I know they would have been proud. Each time I visit China I especially remember their faith in me and their love. I return spiritually replenished.

Finally, I pay tribute to my native country, China, where Traditional Chinese Medicine and Chinese philosophy have been developed and passed down the generations. It is ancient and yet current. Because of it, the Chinese as a nation live healthy lives.

In writing this book, I want to bring the benefits of TCM and its insights into living a healthy life to the attention of a Western audience. Follow these principles and you will be slim and healthy.